Clinical Risk Management in Midwifery
The right to a perfect baby?

Commissioning editor: Mary Seager
Development editor: Caroline Savage
Production controller: Anthony Read
Desk editor: Jackie Holding
Cover designer: Fred Rose

Clinical Risk Management in Midwifery

The right to a perfect baby?

Jo H Wilson MSc (Dist), PGDip, BSc (Hons), MIPD, AIRM, MHSM, RGN, RM, RSCN
Marsh UK Ltd, High West Jesmond, Newcastle upon Tyne

Andrew Symon RGN, RM, MA (Hons), PhD, Clinical Research Fellow (Midwifery)
School of Nursing and Midwifery, University of Dundee

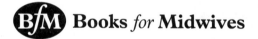 Books *for* Midwives

OXFORD   AUCKLAND   BOSTON   JOHANNESBURG   MELBOURNE   NEW DELHI

Book for Midwives
Butterworth-Heinemann
Linacre House, Jordan Hill, Oxford OX2 8DP
225 Wildwood Avenue, Woburn, MA 01801-2041
A division of Reed Educational and Professional Publishing Ltd

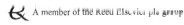 A member of the Reed Elsevier plc group

First published 2002

© Reed Educational and Professional Publishing Ltd 2002

British Library Cataloguing in Publication Data

Wilson, Jo
    Clinical risk management in midwifery: the right to a perfect baby?
    1.   Midwifery – Moral and ethical aspects   2.   Health facilities
    – Risk management   3.   Midwifery – Practice – Law and Legislation
    I.   Title   II.   Symon, Andrew, 1961-
    618.2

ISBN 0 7506 2851 0

For information on all Books for Midwives publications visit our website at www.bh.com/midwifery

Typeset by Keytec Typesetting Ltd, Bridport, Dorset.
Printed and bound in Great Britain by Biddles Ltd, Guildford and King's Lynn

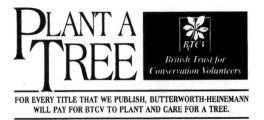

British Trust for
Conservation Volunteers

FOR EVERY TITLE THAT WE PUBLISH, BUTTERWORTH-HEINEMANN
WILL PAY FOR BTCV TO PLANT AND CARE FOR A TREE.

Contents

Preface

Controlling risks in the area of midwifery is a challenge for both medical and midwifery practitioners and also for healthcare risk managers. The midwife is the most senior practitioner at about 70 per cent of all births in the United Kingdom. Historically, litigation cases involving birth injuries have been the most costly; there is a high potential for settlements well in excess of a million pounds due to the cost of providing lifelong care for a handicapped person. High emotions are also associated with injured/damaged babies. There appears to be a public expectation that every pregnancy will be uncomplicated and result in a normal healthy baby; when things go wrong this may lead to the belief that any problems are the result of clinical negligence (this is examined in Chapter 3). It seems as though mothers feel they have the right to a perfect baby, and if the baby is less than perfect then someone is to blame. It is not surprising that anything short of perfection can result in disappointment, complaint and sometimes litigation. In our 'naming, blaming and shaming' society parents may blame practitioners, and practitioners may blame each other.

Although pregnancy is normally an uncomplicated process, many factors can jeopardize the likelihood of the mother giving birth to a normal healthy baby. Identifying these factors and intervening appropriately (managing the known risk) can help increase the chances that a healthy baby will be born. Analysing the risks in obstetrics that most frequently result in claims and developing strong proactive strategies will help to reduce the likelihood of claims arising and will allow for those filed to be more defensible. The aim is to have the best defence in terms of record keeping and communication, and not to practise defensively by trying to 'cover your back' by inappropriate activities. Obstetric practitioners should incorporate their knowledge and skills with proactive risk management and continuous quality improvement strategies in order to promote maternal and fetal wellbeing. A more proactive approach to care management will result in better quality of care and risk management, which will in turn reduce the likelihood of adverse outcomes. For this approach to succeed, it is essential that the care provided by midwives reflects both an understanding of the risks involved, and knowledge, expertise and confidence in applying risk management.

This book focuses on a number of the issues outlined within the case study used in Chapter 1 and on other factors that are essential for effective midwifery care. Chapter 2 looks at the communication and documentation issues, with particular emphasis on the mother being a partner in the delivery of care and the requirement for excellent team working. *The Fifth Annual Report of the Confidential Enquiry into Stillbirths and Deaths in Infancy*, published by the Maternal and Child Health Research Consortium in 1998, identified 95 per cent of critical comments acknowledging failures in three main areas: to recognize that a problem existed, to take appropriate action, and in communication. 'Communication failure' was cited as responsible for 17 per cent of cases with a poor outcome, including poor utilization and non-existence of chain of command and jump call policies. The utilization of maternal records, usage of hand-held records and the use of multidisciplinary pathways of care as part of integrated care management and team working will also be explored.

Chapter 3 looks at the midwife and the legal environment, and includes an introduction to the law of clinical negligence and a discussion of the implications of litigation. Chapter 4 addresses intra- and inter-professional behaviour and communication and the effect they can have on the delivery of care. This includes an examination of autonomy and workplace behaviour, and the role of the midwife as part of the multidisciplinary team.

The book then starts to address the management, supervision and responsibilities for risk management, with Chapter 5 exploring the role of the midwifery manager and supervisor of midwives. It will discuss issues such as: who takes responsibility for managing risk; how to ensure everyone has a role and responsibility; water births and how supervision can help in risk identification; and formulation of agreed strategies. Chapter 6 addresses the role of informed consent and the competent adult, the incompetent adult and the law. It reviews recent cases that have changed practice, and discusses issues such as the rights of the fetus, contraception, and abortion.

The book then starts to address more specific issues, with Chapter 7 discussing the role of genetic counselling and ethical issues. Included in this are the right to opt for termination of pregnancy, and the best use of information and decision-making. It explores how active or passive the woman is in the decision-making process, and the role of the autonomous practitioner in decision-making. Chapter 8 specifically addresses the tools of risk management and their application to midwifery practice, including which tools are the most effective and how to apply them. It also looks at the role and analysis of complaints and clinical incidents, clinical benchmarking, outcome of care, patient satisfaction and changing practice parameters.

We then move onto the views of the mother and her level of involvement in the midwifery system and care delivery processes. Chapter 9 starts to look at the consumer view in Changing Childbirth, the use of birth plans, and the role of groups such as the National Childbirth Trust. It looks at the mother's perception of risks and whether she feels the information she is given and the consultations she has are adequate. Does she feel part of the decision-making process? Chapter 10 considers who the victims of midwifery accidents are, how they are dealt with, whether women should have the expectation of always getting a perfect baby, and who cares for and looks after the midwife.

The book concludes with Chapter 11, which discusses using a proactive and preventative overview to ensure the application of effective risk management and strategies for coping and providing a controlled environment of care. The book provides many practical examples and case studies that will be useful for local application, learning the lessons and sharing good practice. We hope you will enjoy reading this and find it a useful reference book for everyday midwifery practice.

J H Wilson and A Symon

1

Principles of clinical governance

Jo Wilson

Introduction

Most of the elements of clinical governance (Figure 1.1) are not new to good midwives and managers, but the accountability framework brings them together under one umbrella. This provides a protective mechanism for both public and staff, and demonstrates that their local healthcare organizations are actively developing structures to improve quality and standards of maternity care. It is about having efficient and effective systems of communication with staff and patients, and the establishment of robust infrastructures to develop evidence-based quality health care proactively.

Risk management is the lynch pin that pulls together all the different elements of clinical governance. It also pulls together the accountability frameworks and clear reporting mechanisms to meet the Corporate Governance and Controls Assurance requirements.

Clinical governance incorporates a number of processes, including:

- Clinical audit
- Evidence-based practice in daily use supported within the infrastructure

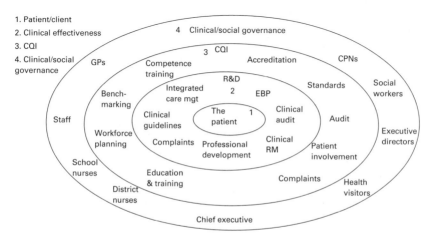

Figure 1.1 The components required for clinical governance.

- Clinical effectiveness
- Clinical risk management with adverse events being detected, openly investigated and lessons learned
- Lessons for improving practice being learned from complaints
- Outcomes of care
- Good quality clinical data being used to monitor clinical care with problems of poor clinical practice being recognized early and dealt with
- Good practice being systematically disseminated within and outside the organization
- Clinical risk reduction programmes of a high standard being in place.

There is an expectation that all midwives should participate fully in audit programmes, including national external audit programmes, such as the *Confidential Enquiries into Maternal Deaths* (*CEMD*) and *Confidential Enquiries into Stillbirths and Deaths in Infancy* (*CESDI*), which are endorsed by the Commission for Health Improvement. Clinical governance places a duty of responsibility on all maternity professionals to ensure that care is satisfactory, consistent and responsive; individuals are responsible for the quality of their midwifery practice as part of professional self-regulation. It will strengthen the current systems of quality assurance based on evaluation of clinical standards (including *Towards Safer Childbirth*), better utilization of evidence-based practice and learning lessons from poor performance. The clinical governance framework builds upon professional self-regulation and performance review; it takes account of existing systems of quality control and includes all activity and information for quality improvements. It is based upon partnership, and driven by performance based on efficiency, effectiveness and excellence.

The clinical governance processes in midwifery care include:

- Improvements in clinical quality that identify and build on good practice and are integrated with the overall organizational quality improvement programmes
- The systematic dissemination of good practice
- The existence of clinical risk reduction programmes
- Professional self-regulation and assessment (including the development of clinical leadership skills)
- The presence of evidence-based practice systems
- The detection and open investigation of adverse events, near misses and incidents
- The learning of lessons from the above
- Complaints being dealt with positively and the information being used to improve the organization and delivery of care
- The collection of high quality performance measurement data to monitor clinical care and support professionals in delivering high standards of care
- Dealing appropriately with poor clinical performance so as to minimize harm to patients and staff
- Supporting staff in their duty to report concerns about colleagues' professional conduct and performance (procedures need to be developed to support the individual in remedying the situation)
- Continuing professional development through lifelong learning aligned with clinical governance principles.

Clinical risk management is a synergy between risk management, quality and the law. It also allows for the establishment of multidisciplinary standards of care and best practice guidelines to enhance professional development of maternity services. The changes in maternity care, with much higher expectations from mothers, greater clarity of roles and responsibilities of clinicians, and the emphasis on devolving decision-making as close to the mother as possible, are intended to affect the entire performance of maternity care.

Near miss and incident reporting

In the Department of Health Report *An Organization with a Memory* (DoH, 2000) the clear message portrayed is that lessons are not learned when things go wrong. This certainly applies to the maternity services; the successive *CESDI* reports (e.g. MCHRC, 1998, 2000) have identified very similar instances of poor practice. Many of the identified poor outcomes could have been avoided if only lessons had been properly learned. Clinical governance can provide a powerful imperative to focus on tackling adverse healthcare events. To support this process and to modernize the approach to learning from failures, the Department of Health report outlines four key areas that need to be tackled:

1. Unified mechanisms for reporting and analysis when things go wrong
2. A more open culture, in which errors or service failures can be reported and discussed
3. Mechanisms for ensuring that where lessons are identified, the necessary changes are put into practice
4. A much wider appreciation of the value of the systems approach in preventing, analysing and learning from errors.

In near miss and incident reporting, all near misses should be viewed as free lessons and incidents as opportunities to improve the quality of service provision (Wilson, 1998). Incident reporting, investigation and follow-up are considered a minimum, level one standard of the Clinical Negligence Scheme for Trusts (CNST; Wilson, 1997), alongside the clinical complaints procedure, which is a means of assessing areas where improvements need to be made. The Clinical Negligence and Other Risks Indemnity Scheme (CNORIS), which is the Scottish equivalent, has the same requirements. The reporting of near misses is also important, as we can learn from these and put systems in place to reduce the likelihood of their recurrence. Having an open, just, honest and participative organization that is open to improving processes and systems of maternity care is a big step towards having staff committed to quality and getting things right.

Near miss, incident and indicator recording and reporting are a cornerstone of any quality and risk management system. Yet in the Department of Health report the evidence suggests that around 850 000 adverse events, at probably in excess of a cost of £2 billion, occur every year in the NHS. Case studies within the report highlight the consequences of weaknesses in the ability of the NHS to learn lessons. The *CEMD* and *CESDI* have helped to identify certain major critical incidents and have assisted in producing clinical guidelines and protocols to minimize recurrence. An area that will prove to be much more important and more proactive will be the identification of near misses, which will help clinicians to recognize why and how complications may occur and how they can be prevented, thereby reducing the exposure to adverse incidents, complaints and clinical negligence claims.

Understanding the causes of failure

An Organization with a Memory (DoH, 2000) deals with the causes of failure and a number of different perspectives from the research undertaken within this area. Human error can be viewed in two different ways; as a person-centred approach and as a systems approach. Professor Brian Toft (1992) has undertaken much work on these different approaches in industry, and the approaches have been applied to health care by Professor James Reason (1997).

Individual failures

As demonstrated by Toft (1992), Reason (1997), and Wilson (1998), the person-centred approach is the more dominant tradition in healthcare settings, with the focus on individual behaviour – 'naming, blaming and shaming'. Healthcare professionals use it on each other and patients now also generally use it, believing that if something goes wrong or if there is an unexpected outcome, someone must be to blame. In research undertaken by the authors (Wilson and Tingle, 1999), most incidents involved a systems failure. There are usually several factors combined that lead up to the incident or near miss, with a number of quality failures that lead up to the adverse event. It is rare that there is only one person who is responsible, as there is usually a sequence of events, and generally the blame that is applied is due more to matters of opinion than matters of fact.

Research undertaken by Professor John Øvretveit (1998) suggests that 85 per cent of adverse incidents are due to organizational failures and 15 per cent to individual failures. The individual failures include inattention to detail, lapses of memory, negligence, forgetfulness, and carelessness. This was corroborated by the authors, who agreed with the overall findings on remedial action – which often suited the hierarchical management style – with 98 per cent concentration on the individual failures and only 2 per cent on the organizational failures.

Systems failures

With most incidents being caused by organizational failures, the *Organization with a Memory* report (DoH, 2000) favours the systems approach and having the right people in place to implement the processes and systems of care delivery. The systems approach takes a holistic view on the issues of failures and looks at complex organizations with ill-defined responsibilities, policies and procedures, and multifarious factors that come together, where some degree of error is inevitable. All organizations operating in hazardous circumstances tend to develop barriers, defences and safeguards that become interposed between the source of the hazard and the potential victims, or the losses that occur should that risk become realized.

Professor Reason's model (see Figure 1.2; also DoH, 2000) tries to analyse near misses and incidents that occur in healthcare settings by looking at the sequence of events that lead up to early detection (a near miss) or when an

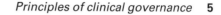

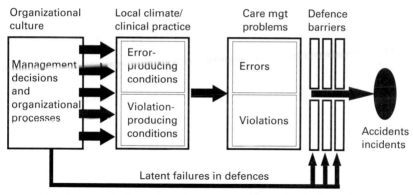

| Organizational culture | Local climate/ clinical practice | Care mgt problems | Defence barriers |

Figure 1.2 Serious accidents don't just happen (reprinted with kind permission from Professor J. Reason, 1997).

accident or incident actually occurs. It can then be used to look back at the conditions in which staff were working and the organizational context in which the near miss or incident/accident occurred.

The model is best understood if studied from right to left, looking at the situations that led to a breakdown in the defence barriers. This breakdown in the defence barriers is often described as the domino effect or, more appropriately, the Swiss cheese model. This likens the events to having all defences in place at all times to prevent hazards or losses, whereas in reality the defences are more like Swiss cheese (Figure 1.3), being full of holes. However, unlike the holes in the cheese, the gaps in system defences are continuously opening, shutting and

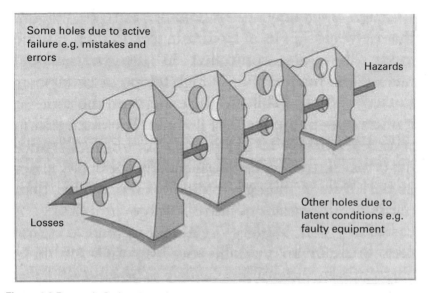

Figure 1.3 Reason's Swiss cheese model of accident causation (adapted with kind permission from Professor J. Reason, 1997).

shifting position. These shifts in position are due to active failures and latent conditions.

System failure types

Behind these error-producing conditions may lie a further set of wider organizational problems such as a conflict between profit and safety, inadequate communication and deficient training. They include:

- Incompatible goals between different staffing levels within the organization
- No shared goals from the Trust Board downwards with shared values and objectives
- Structural (organizational) deficiencies that do not have a corporate influence and a shared commitment and vision
- Inadequate communication, with no clear strategy, information sharing or two-way process to ensure involvement at all levels
- Poor planning and scheduling, leading to frustrations, delays and negative effects on patient care (such as being kept 'nil by mouth' for long periods), and patient complaints due to indecision and staff uncertainty
- Inadequate control and monitoring, with lack of leadership in tackling issues, resulting in staff frustration and demotivation
- Design failures, with lack of consultation and involvement of users who have to suffer the consequences (including patient dissatisfaction)
- Deficient training, with inadequate preparation, ongoing education and development to help staff cope with eventualities
- Inadequate maintenance management, with poor facilities and equipment and lack of ownership leading to sick building syndrome and feelings that no one cares about the environment or the people working within it.

The first step is to identify the active failures whose actions can have immediate adverse consequences.

Active failures

An Organization with a Memory (DoH, 2000) discusses active failures that include unsafe acts or omissions committed by those at the 'sharp end' of the systems (e.g. pilots, air-traffic controllers, obstetricians, midwives and nurses). These can be caused by memory lapses and mistakes through ignorance or misreading the situation, slips or failures (such as picking up the wrong syringe), forgetting to carry out a procedure, or even violations (deviations from safe practices, procedures or standards of care). Rarely, there can be deliberate departures from safe operating practices, procedures or standards due to conflict with management.

Examples of active failures types include the following:

- The significance of changes on a CTG trace may not be given sufficient weight, which can result in a prolonged labour and a compromised baby
- Inappropriate use of syntocinon, particularly when fetal compromise is suspected
- Inappropriate decision-making by senior staff, which may occur when they are asked to attend but only receive partial information.

Latent conditions

These arise from fallible decisions, often taken by people not directly involved in the workplace (Reason, 1997). They can lie dormant in the workplace for long periods before combining with local factors and active failures to penetrate, break down or bypass defences. They provide the conditions (outlined by Wilson and Tingle, 1999) in which unsafe acts occur:

- High workload, time pressures, fatigue
- Inadequate knowledge, ability or experience
- Inadequate supervision or instruction
- A stressful environment; rapid change within an organization
- Inadequate communication and documentation
- Poor maintenance of equipment and buildings
- Incompatible goals, which can cause conflict.

Latent failures are always present, and they can be identified or removed prior to causing an accident or incident. The culture and core beliefs of the organization and values of the staff need to change to deal with such issues on a proactive basis.

Examples of latent condition failure types include the following:

- No clear demarcation of roles and responsibilities, and no agreed lines of communication
- No chain of command or 'jump call policy' to follow in a crisis
- Staff who have received inadequate training (e.g. in CTG interpretation)
- Poorly maintained equipment, which can lead to practitioners assuming that the equipment is at fault when in fact there is significant fetal compromise.

Principles of safety: human factors approaches

The analysis here is much more focused on the organizational causes of near misses and incidents, rather than on individuals. The root causes of adverse events, including all near misses and incidents, lie in failures of some or all of the following (Reason, 1997):

- Adequate communication
- Meticulous, contemporaneous documentation
- Adequate levels of supervision; responsibility and accountability
- Availability of up-to-date policies, procedures and guidelines
- Safe up-to-date clinical practice
- Reasonable workload levels, including appropriateness of staffing and resources
- Use of locum/bank/temporary staff
- Safe organizational practices with adequate human resource and people management
- Health and safety at work
- Education and training for all staff
- Safe systems of work
- Performance management and staff appraisal systems, and having healthy staff who are fit to practise.

As outlined by Wilson and Tingle (1999), these tools of risk modification are designed to promote proactive risk management and to concentrate on providing a controlled environment of care in which the multidisciplinary team can minimize and/or eliminate the causes of identified risk failures. Having these safeguards in place will assist professionals in the audit and evaluation of care.

What does this tell us about our systems?

The *Organization with a Memory* report (DoH, 2000) deals with how an ongoing analysis of near misses and incidents will bring rich detail regarding the evolution of adverse outcomes and their underlying causes. Awareness of the nature, causes and incidence of failures is a vital component of prevention; and prevention is cheaper than cure.

It is possible to identify common themes or characteristics in failures, which should be of use in helping to predict and prevent further adverse events. Seventy per cent of healthcare incidents are preventable, and all errors can be minimized (DoH, 2000). It is essential then that these lessons are learned with appropriate practice, policy and system, to minimize recurrence.

The findings of the expert group in the *Organization with a Memory* report highlight changes that all NHS organizations can start to implement – and many already have – before national action takes place. The group supports using the systems approach to take a holistic view of failure within organizations. This, coupled with focusing on both error management and error prevention, is an important part of developing organizations that can provide ongoing learning and improvements in quality and safety.

The NHS must use an active learning approach to help develop an 'informed culture' where safety is an important feature. This also creates an environment in which people can learn from and respond to failures. Everyone knows that changing the culture of the organization is hard work, but it is possible. Some of the actions needed to develop an informed culture will already have been undertaken by many organizations (Wilson, 1999), and include:

- Raising the awareness of the costs of not taking risk seriously
- Priority given to reporting and feedback to staff, with tracking and trending and actions taken to prevent recurrence
- Training, to avoid failure to identify serious events due to lack of awareness
- Correction of the wrong systems and processes
- Focusing on near misses as well as incidents
- Ensuring that concerns can be reported without fear, threats of disciplinary and punitive actions
- Using external input to stimulate learning
- Giving a high profile lead on the issues, and demonstrating commitment of the Trust Board and senior medical and nursing clinicians.

Learning from near misses and incidents needs to take place on three levels of organizational learning. The first level means that individuals and the maternity unit involved in the particular incident can each draw their own lessons from it. At the second level, more general lessons, across all maternity units, can be drawn from an analysis of the factors surrounding the incident. Finally, some learning can take place simply as a result of being made aware that a particular event has taken place. Learning the lessons from near misses and incidents is a key component of clinical governance and improvements in standards of maternity care, and will be an essential part of delivering the organizational quality strategy.

This includes ensuring that factors of causation and analysis are recognized and shared, with a preventative focus looking at the conditions and systems of work. Each maternity unit needs to develop tools to analyse systematically its own safety performance and to have a framework of background conditions that preclude risk and unsafe practice, which can be monitored to assess the health of the organization and its vital signs. This is a proactive and essential component of any risk and quality management system, and must be embedded within the organization.

Case study

The following case study, which draws on a real case, highlights several of the issues covered already in this chapter. It draws out some of the lessons of clinical risk management. The names and hospital details presented are fictitious in order to protect the individuals involved in the case.

Mrs Bruce versus Rosehill Trust

Mrs Bruce was an 18-year-old primigravida. Her antenatal history had been relatively uneventful; she suffered from early morning sickness for the first 12 weeks, but was well for the rest of her pregnancy. Her last menstrual period was stated to have been in the second week in December, and her expected date of delivery was 18 September. On booking into the Trust for shared care, she was approximately 20 weeks pregnant.

At 1610 hours on 26 August, in her 36th week of pregnancy, Mrs Bruce was admitted to the Rosehill Trust hospital in early labour. Uterine contractions had commenced 2 hours prior to admission and were 10 minutes apart; her membranes were intact. On examination, her cervix was found to be 75 per cent effaced and 2 cm dilated, and the fetal head was above the ischial spines (at level −5).

At 1830 hours an external monitor was applied for a 30-minute period. The tracing is of very poor quality and appears to represent mostly artefact. At 1911 hours, Dr Sainsbury, the obstetric registrar caring for the patient, performed an artificial rupture of membranes, and meconium-stained amniotic fluid was noted.

At 1920 hours, continuous external monitoring was commenced; not until 2015 hours was an internal scalp electrode applied. The vaginal examination at this time revealed the cervix to be fully effaced and 4–5 cm dilated, and the fetal head deeply engaged. The baseline fetal heart rate (FHR) was 180 bpm (beats per minute), with variable decelerations evident almost immediately. At 2040 hours there was a prolonged late FHR deceleration to 70 bpm. Dr Sainsbury was present, and Mrs Bruce was turned onto her side and given oxygen. FHR variability was reduced, and subtle late decelerations continued to occur throughout the remainder of her labour. Dr Roberts, the neonatal registrar, was asked to see the patient. He then left and was not called back until after the delivery.

At 2130 hours, Dr Sainsbury examined Mrs Bruce and noted that her cervix was fully dilated; soon afterwards he commenced a syntocinon infusion, and Mrs Bruce was given an opiate injection at 2144 hours. At 2234 hours a male infant, Marc, weighing 2.83 kg (6 lb 4 oz), was born spontaneously. His Apgar scores were 3 at 1 minute and 5 at 5 minutes. The baby was heavily meconium stained, pale and atonic, and did not breathe. His airways were cleared using suction, and he was intubated and given oxygen. Narcan was administered approximately 5 minutes after delivery.

Marc was then admitted to the special care baby unit (SCBU) at 2255 hours and later transferred to the regional neonatal intensive care unit (NICU) at 0230 hours. He was suffering from haemolytic anaemia due to an ABO incompatibility, for which an exchange transfusion was performed. A chest X-ray was undertaken and revealed no meconium aspiration but a mild left lower lobe consolidation. Marc's respiratory status improved rapidly, and he was nursed in room air by day six. He fed well, his parents participated in most of his care, and he was thriving and behaving normally. An EEG on the day prior to discharge was normal, and the consultant neonatologist was very optimistic about his long-term prognosis. Marc was discharged on 6 September, at 11 days of age.

He and his parents were seen in the paediatric outpatients department by Dr Roberts, neonatal registrar, on 16 September. Marc was then 3 weeks old, and he was found to have a normal physical and neurological examination. Marc is now 5 years old and is alleged to have cerebral palsy.

Medical expert opinion

Dr Lavin, a consultant obstetrician at another Trust, reviewed the case and gave an opinion to the defendants' solicitors. He was very critical of the care given to this mother during labour and delivery. He felt that the Rosehill Trust was negligent in not calling in the patient's consultant, Dr Thomas, or notifying him of the complications during labour. On the basis of the meconium staining, poor FHR variability and persistent late decelerations, he criticized Dr Sainsbury for not recognizing the possibility of fetal compromise. He also criticized the administration of syntocinon at 2145 hours, and stated that Dr Roberts should have been present at the delivery.

Dr Lavin was critical of the midwives for allowing all of this to occur without alerting their midwifery supervisor or the consultant to the problems, and of the hospital for not having fetal scalp sampling available. Lastly, he stated the baby was inadequately oxygenated after delivery.

Risk management issues

The factors that contribute to perinatal morbidity and mortality are numerous. Almost 20 per cent of all pregnant women fall into the high-risk categories, and these high-risk factors (outlined in Table 1.1) account for 50 per cent of perinatal deaths and are associated with seven obstetrical conditions (Jensen *et al.*, 1981). The seven stated conditions are:

1. Breech presentation
2. Premature separation of the normally implanted placenta
3. Pre-eclampsia or eclampsia
4. Multiple pregnancy
5. Pyelonephritis

Table 1.1 Maternal clinical high-risk factors

Maternal past history:
- Hereditary abnormalities
- Preterm delivery
- Congenital blood anomalies
- Teenage pregnancy
- Drug abuse/addiction
- No antenatal care
- Maternal age > 35 years
- Exposure to rubella and cytomegalovirus
- More than five pregnancies > 35 years
- Prolonged infertility or hormone treatment
- Stressful or dangerous events during pregnancy (e.g. critical accident or radiation exposure)
- Heavy cigarette smoking
- Conception within 2 months of previous delivery

Diagnosis of any of the following:
- Complications of pre-eclampsia, eclampsia, multiple pregnancy, hydramnios
- Height under 147 cm (4 ft 10 in)
- Minimum or no weight gain during pregnancy
- Pregnancy > 42 weeks' gestation
- Abnormal fetal growth
- Abnormal presentation of fetus (e.g. breech or non-engaged presenting part at term)
- Rhesus/ABO incompatibility

---

6. Hydramnios
7. Premature labour.

Neonatal brain damage can be due to the following, either alone or in combination (Nelson, 1987):

- Hypoxia
- Ischaemia (low blood pressure and low blood flow)
- Haemorrhages – spontaneous or traumatic
- Apnoea
- Hypoglycaemia (low blood sugar level)
- Kernicterus (excessive bilirubin level in the blood)
- Infection (e.g. meningitis)
- Seizures (which complicate and exacerbate other pathological processes)
- Hydrocephalus.

While it is believed that there is only a small proportion of neonatal brain damage that is the direct result of obstetric clinical malpractice or negligence, there are sometimes conflicting views regarding causation (there is much research ongoing in this area, looking particularly at the condition of the placenta). In order to secure compensation, a claimant must show that the negligence of a practitioner (whether through act or omission) either caused or materially contributed to the damage. The requirements of the law of medical negligence are set out in more detail in Chapter 3. Even if the defendants concede that the standard of care was inadequate, they may maintain that the damage the baby suffered occurred before the birth process, and that therefore it was not caused by the actions or omissions of the practitioner. The claimants will attempt to prove that the defendants' negligence before or during the birth process has resulted in the baby suffering diffuse brain injury; they will argue that this injury is not the result of some congenital defect or early pregnancy asphyxial insult.

Obstetrical claims, especially for brain-damaged babies, represent a major area of financial loss to the Trusts. In 1989, UK indemnity payments by speciality showed obstetrics to be the highest at 23.7 per cent (MPS, 1989). In 1997 the contingent liability for obstetrics by the value of cases was 70 per cent, and by number of claims, 27 per cent (NHS Litigation Authority). The NHS Litigation Authority (NHS LA) also gives a figure of £242 782 343 as the total claims paid out for obstetrics since 1 April 1995 – 64 per cent of claims in all specialities. The clinical maternal high-risk factors are highlighted in Table 1.1, and the risk factors requiring further evaluation in Table 1.2.

In the case study discussed, some of the issues the practitioners should have been alerted to and acted upon were the meconium-stained liquor, the abnormalities in the cardiotocograph (CTG), and the length of the second stage of labour. There should always be an appropriately trained practitioner (this may be a neonatologist or paediatrician) present at all deliveries where there is any meconium staining and/or significant fetal heart decelerations. It always seems easier to criticize when looking in on other people mishaps, and to comment on what action should have been taken, especially when all the circumstances are not known. It is vitally important after any critical clinical incidents that the multidisciplinary team reviews the case and identifies the appropriate lessons. Table 1.3 contains the criteria for perinatal services clinical audit review, which should be undertaken by the multidisciplinary team on a regular basis.

Table 1.2 Risk factors requiring further evaluation

Maternal history of:
- Prolonged rupture of membranes
- Abnormal presentation and delivery
- Prolonged, difficult or precipitous labour
- Prolapsed cord

Birth asphyxia suggested by:
- Fetal heart rate fluctuations
- Meconium staining
- Fetal acidosis (pH below 7.2)
- Apgar scores less than 7, especially at 5 minutes
- Preterm birth < 37 weeks
- Post-term birth > 42 weeks
- Small or large gestational infants
- Any respiratory distress or apnoea
- Obvious congenital anomalies
- Convulsions, limpness or sucking/swallowing difficulties
- Distension, vomiting or both
- Anaemia (Hb > 15 gm) or bleeding tendency
- Jaundiced in first 24 hours, or bilirubin level > 15 mg/l

Table 1.3 Perinatal services: clinical audit risk management review criteria

Cause for review	Review criteria
Maternal deaths	Documented evaluation of maternal risk factors and referrals made
	Appropriate identification and management of hypertension or bleeding
	Uterine monitoring where syntocinon or other drugs were used
Antepartum fetal deaths > 24 weeks	Documented evaluation of maternal and fetal risk factors and referrals made
	Documentation of timely and appropriate antenatal testing
	Documentation of accurate interpretation of antenatal tests
Neonatal deaths and intrapartum fetal deaths	Documentation of fetal wellbeing on admission, labour and delivery
	Documented reassessments of the fetus
	Appropriate monitoring where syntocinon or other drugs were used
	Documentation of the resuscitation of a live-born infant
LSCS for fetal indication not started within 30 minutes	Documentation of timely and appropriate assessments of the fetus
	Documentation of the decision to proceed to Caesarean section
Neonates > 34 weeks transferred to a NNU	Documentation of the delivery room staff anticipating the needs of the neonate and planning appropriately for them, e.g. transfer
	Documentation of fetal wellbeing on admission, in labour and at delivery
	Documented reassessment of the fetus
	Documentation of the resuscitation

We can lessen the possibility of clinical negligence by addressing our responsibility to the patient, to her care and treatment, and to the care and treatment of the neonate by providing the best possible level of care. There is a synergy between risk management, quality and good obstetric care, and we need to get this right in order to practise what we preach. Bear in mind that we live in a society that seems to believe anything less than a perfect result is indicative of clinical negligence.

Healthcare organizations, especially in potentially high-risk specialities like obstetrics, need to demonstrate their high levels of achievement and commitment to continuous quality improvements. The main purpose of healthcare delivery is to secure, through the resources available, the greatest possible maintenance of and improvement in the physical and mental health of the population, and the wellbeing of the mother and her baby. Achieving clinical quality and effective risk management is the aim of every midwife, so it may seem surprising that there is apparently so much variation in practice between hospitals, maternity units and even individuals, all trying to deliver the same kind of service. Some local customization is of course desirable, but the variations in both quality of care and quality of delivery of care would suggest that many of the principles that should underpin any quality service are not always addressed. In the Fifth Annual Report of the *Confidential Enquiry into Stillbirths and Deaths in Infancy* (MCHRC, 1998), over 77 per cent of intra-partum deaths are criticized for sub-optimal care; alternative management 'would have made a difference' to the outcome in 52 per cent of cases, and 'might' have helped in another 25 per cent. The reasons for this are complex, but may relate to an historic narrowness in the training of midwifery and medical professionals; failures of midwives and doctors to work together, an inability to implement change; fears of failure and threats to clinical autonomy and clinical freedom due to lack of evidence-based practice, and a poor record in effective teamworking.

Clinical governance within the healthcare organization provides a clear framework for the achievement of quality improvement (Wilson, 1999). Quality in this context means clinical care as well as customer/client care, and getting things right first time and every time; risk management in terms of avoiding the potential for unwanted outcomes and getting things right every time. Clinical governance encompasses all the processes needed to achieve the highest quality midwifery practice possible within available resources. Clinical governance represents a major opportunity for midwifery professionals, as it gives them the authority they need to make the health service work more effectively (Wilson, 1999).

References

Department of Health (2000). *An Organization with a Memory*. HMSO.

Jensen, M. *et al*. (1981) *Maternity Care*, 3rd edn. CV Mosby Co.

Maternal and Child Health Research Consortium (1998). *Confidential Enquiry into Stillbirths and Deaths in Infancy*, 5th Report. MCHRC.

Maternal and Child Health Research Consortium (2000). *Confidential Enquiry into Stillbirths and Deaths in Infancy*, 7th Report. MCHRC.

Medical Protection Society (1989). *Annual Report*. MPS.

Nelson, R. (1987). *Textbook of Paediatrics*. Churchill Livingstone.

Øvretveit, J. (1998). *Health Service Quality*. Brunel University.

Reason, J. (1997). *Managing the Risk of Organizational Accidents*. Ashgate.

Toft, B. (1992). The failure of hindsight. *Disaster Prevention and Management*, **1(3)**, 213–17.

Vincent, C., Taylor-Adams, S. and Stanhope, N. (1998). Framework for analysing risk and safety in clinical medicine. *Br. Med. J.*, **316**, 1154–7.

Wilson, J. (1997). The Clinical Negligence Scheme for Trusts. *Br. J. Nursing*, **6(20)**, 1166–7.

Wilson, J. (1998). Incident reporting. *Br. J. Nursing*, **7(11)**, 670–71.

Wilson, J. (1999). The route to clinical governance. *Healthcare Risk Report*, **5(4)**, 16–18.

Wilson, J. and Tingle, J. (1999). *Clinical Risk Modification: A Route to Clinical Governance*. Butterworth-Heinemann.

2

Clinical risk modification – a collaborative approach to midwifery care

Jo Wilson

Introduction

Patients' expectations have risen markedly in the last decade, as has the quality and standard of care provided in general. Patients and the public expect the same level of service and quality assurances from health care as they receive from other industries such as hotel chains, department stores and travel services. The UK government is aware of these rising expectations and patient anxieties and concerns with healthcare delivery; hence the implementation of the healthcare reforms (DoH, 1997) in modernizing the NHS to restore public confidence in the service. The government made quality of care a key issue by legislating for it under the Health Act 1999. A statutory duty of quality is placed on all NHS Trusts and Primary Care Trusts, and this duty will operate alongside the duty of care already owed to patients at common law. This is covered in detail in Chapter 3. All Trusts must establish plans for the systematic monitoring of quality and appropriateness of patient care, as well as effective clinical risk management systems to meet corporate and clinical governance requirements. This will include the identification of deviations from established standards of care, and evidence-based practice, in patient injuries and other situations that reflect potential exposure to civil litigation.

Understanding clinical risks in midwifery care

Pregnancy and delivery are anxious periods for many women because of ill-founded fears and misinformation, and some disorders of pregnancy can be aggravated by anxiety. Although pregnancy may be complicated, serious problems are relatively uncommon, and many believe that the public has an expectation that pregnancies and labours will be straightforward – in other words, that people have the right to a perfect baby. This often leads to the belief that any unexpected problems are a result of mistakes and professional errors by staff who do not work well as teams and have poor communication skills. Since the safety of the woman and her baby is paramount in all aspects of maternity care, it is important that all midwives have a good understanding of clinical risk management, that they actively participate in implementing safe practices, and that they act to prevent adverse outcomes.

Although pregnancy is normally an uncomplicated process, many factors can jeopardize the likelihood of the mother giving birth to a normal healthy baby. Identifying these factors and intervening appropriately, through good clinical risk management, can help ensure that a healthy baby will be born. This clinical risk management needs to be much more part of a systematic approach in evaluating both individual and team practices in a more formalized way to learn from near misses and failures. The maternity team must work closely together to identify those women who may have a greater likelihood of pregnancy complications. Effective monitoring and evaluation of maternal care will minimize serious complications. Accurate and complete record keeping of these evaluations and interventions is critical for continuity of care and for providing the best defence if questions about care later arise. It is essential that whenever care is provided there is easy access to maternal records, whether they are 'hand held' (by the mother) or kept by the midwives and doctors. By careful monitoring in the antenatal period, disorders can be identified quickly, and prompt treatment may eliminate or reduce the problem.

Clinical risk modification in midwifery

The tools of clinical risk modification are designed to be proactive and to concentrate on helping the multidisciplinary team to minimize or eliminate the cause of the identified potential risk. They should be locally owned and controlled to assist professionals in the audit and evaluation of care. They also serve as a change management mechanism for the midwifery organization striving towards the best outcomes. This incorporates having clear mechanisms for risk-prone areas such as dealing with cardiotocograph (CTG) interpretation, and staff awareness and understanding of obstetric emergencies (e.g. shoulder dystocia). It includes contingency plans with regular drills and skills training to test their effectiveness.

Table 2.1 demonstrates the areas that need to be focused upon in order to achieve clinical risk modification, and helps to identify areas where the appropriate processes and systems are not clearly defined or where short cuts are allowed or forced to take place due to workforce or organizational problems. It highlights the issue of staff not being aware of their roles and responsibilities and being forced or pressurized to work beyond their skills and competency levels without the necessary education and training.

It is essential within midwifery practice that the chain of command is well understood. A 'jump call' policy (see Figure 2.1) can help staff to cope with all

Table 2.1 Why do risks occur?

- System failures
- Short cuts
- Communication breakdowns
- Ill-defined responsibilities
- Inadequately trained staff
- Inadequate policies, guidelines and procedures
- Poor inter-agency or inter-departmental working
- Dishonesty

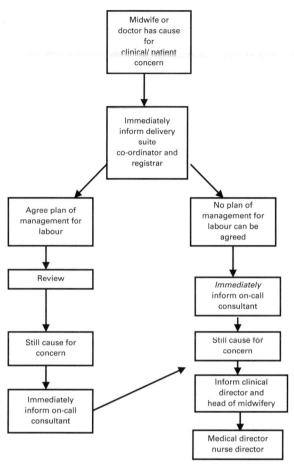

Figure 2.1 Jump call procedure in the delivery suite.

situations when conflicts between care providers arise. However, written policies do not always exist, and in one midwifery unit there were two baby deaths and one cerebral palsy case due to conflict between a midwife and a middle grade doctor (Wilson, 1999). It is not enough to agree a process; the policies must be written down and agreed by the team. A clear chain of command is essential so that staff know when to contact a more senior person if they need to discuss management decisions about which they are not happy. This should be illustrated by a clear flow diagram that outlines the policy and chain of command (see Figure 2.2).

Jump call procedure in the delivery suite

1. Any midwife or doctor who has cause for clinical concern with a labouring woman in their care *must immediately inform* the delivery suite co-ordinator (DSC) and the registrar if the problem is not outside the DSC's scope of practice.

2. A plan of management for labour should be agreed between the midwife/ doctor, the DSC and, if appropriate, the registrar.
3. If a plan of management for labour cannot be agreed or it is not appropriate to 'wait and see', the on-call consultant *must be informed immediately.*
4. If a plan of management for labour cannot be agreed or it is not appropriate to 'wait and see', then the Clinical director and/or the Head of midwifery *must be informed immediately.*
5. If a plan of management for labour cannot be agreed or it is not appropriate to 'wait and see', the Medical director and/or the Nurse director *must be informed immediately.*
6. If a plan of management for labour is agreed, there must be a *timescale* for review of the plan.
7. If at review there is still cause for clinical concern, the on-call consultant *must be informed immediately.*
8. If at review with the on-call consultant there is still cause for clinical concern, the Clinical director and Head of midwifery *must be informed immediately.*

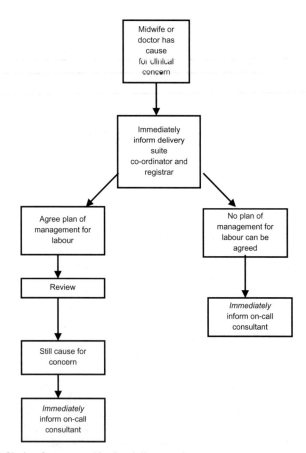

Figure 2.2 Chain of command in the delivery suite.

9. If at review there is still cause for clinical concern, and patient care is thought to be still at risk or care is being compromised, the Medical and/or Nurse director *must be informed immediately.*

Chain of command in the delivery suite

1. Any midwife or doctor who has cause for clinical concern with a labouring woman in their care *must immediately inform* the delivery suite co-ordinator (DSC) and the registrar if the problem is not outside the DSC's scope of practice.
2. A plan of management for labour should be agreed between the midwife/doctor, the DSC and, if appropriate, the registrar.
3. If a plan of management for labour cannot be agreed or it is not appropriate to 'wait and see', the on-call consultant *must be informed immediately.*
4. If a plan of management for labour is agreed, there must be a *timescale* for review of the plan.
5. If at review there is still cause for clinical concern, the on-call consultant *must be informed immediately.*

According to claims and incident analysis (Wilson, 1999), there are some key problem areas, where things do go wrong. In order to achieve clinical risk modification we need to have risk identification and control in these processes. Again they cover communication, documentation and consent to treatment (this will be covered in Chapter 6). Supervision of junior and trainee staff, including locums and new staff, is an important risk and quality issue in terms of the need for appropriate induction, orientation, education and ongoing training. Too often staff are left to undertake procedures where they do not have the skills, competence or supervision to carry them out safely. They may feel pressurized or afraid to ask or admit they have not done this before. One of the problem areas is when junior doctors are left unsupervised when their senior colleagues are on study leave or holiday, and no one is nominated to undertake their supervision. All staff practising in midwifery care must have the knowledge, skills, confidence, judgement and attitude to perform all care provision to the minimum standards of safer childbirth.

Clinical risk management issues in maternity units

Some specialities are more risky than others according to their claims profile, with obstetrics carrying the highest risk (Law *et al.*, 1996). An analysis by the author of 401 closed claims (identified between March 1993 and July 1995 from a number of sources, including law journals, firms of solicitors, the General Medical Council and some hospitals), is shown in Table 2.2.

Table 2.3 shows data published in *The Sunday Times* in October 1995 by The Scottish Office, regarding 1185 cases that were open in August 1995.

The cost of litigation is continuing to rise in the UK, and the costs associated with the 401 closed claims listed in Table 2.2 resulted in a total of £23 909 596 awarded, with an average of £59 182 per claim and a median of £8 000 (these figures do not include legal costs). Of these awards, 38 per cent of the total costs were accounted for by obstetrics and gynaecology. Obstetric claims alone cost

Table 2.2 The relative risks of medical specialities: UK experience

Speciality	No. of claims	Percentage of total
Obstetric	101	25.2
Gynaecology	57	14.2
Orthopaedics	49	12.2
Anaesthetics	43	10.7
Accident and emergency	30	7.5
General surgery	28	7
Others	93	23.2
Total	*401*	100

Table 2.3 The relative risks of medical specialities: Scottish Office

Speciality	Relative risk (%)
Obstetrics and gynaecology	27
Accident and emergency	17
Orthopaedics	13
General surgery	12
Other areas	31
Total	100

£6.87m, with claims from Gynaecology amounting to £2.4m. The average cost for an obstetric claim in this analysis was £68 080 (£42 335 for a gynaecological claim), clearly demonstrating this to be an expensive speciality. Recent figures from the NHS Litigation Authority (Sanderson, 1998) give a figure of over £242m paid out for obstetrics claims since 1 April 1995, accounting for 64 per cent of the total cost from all specialities.

A further analysis of the 401 claims examined by the author revealed the following factors specific to the obstetric allegations:

- A high proportion of the claims involved death or brain damage in the infant allegedly due to birth asphyxia and/or inappropriate delivery
- Inadequate fetal monitoring (including care, action taken and the recording of CTGs and pH levels of the fetus) leading to delays in instigating treatments and interventions
- Delays in performing Caesarean sections due to a number of factors, including inadequate training and supervision of junior medical staff; inadequately defined chain of command, with the consequent fear of upsetting teamworking or allowing arguments to become personal; lack of experienced personnel available to perform the emergency operation; and lack of theatre facilities or staff to perform the procedure
- Delays in involving senior medical staff due to fears about not being able to cope or the attitude or inappropriate responses of some senior practitioners
- Intra-operative problems included equipment failures due to lack of maintenance, or poor training in usage; there was not always backup equipment if something malfunctioned or became unsafe.

Other factors that were also seen in non-obstetric claims were:

- Inconsistent and poor record keeping
- Incomplete or missing documentation
- The inability to locate relevant members of staff
- Lack of information and consent
- Unhelpful remarks
- Lack of explanations and 'saying sorry'. (Wilson, 1999)

Very often it is through analysing what has gone wrong that we can make better provision for the future. Risk modification relies in part on our understanding of what has happened in the past, and one of the ways in which this is done is through the use of clinical indicators.

Use of clinical indicators in midwifery/obstetric care

One of the ways by which we understand risk is to record when things go wrong. Reports into poor clinical outcomes (for example MCHRC, 1998, 2000) or an examination of legal claims can suggest areas that need special care and attention. This can be proactive, i.e. existing data on poor outcomes can provide us with 'early warning signs' so that women at higher risk of certain clinical outcomes can receive appropriate management, or retrospective, in which case sensitive investigation and explanation are applied. Such data also give us a comparative data source with other specialities or Trusts. This encourages the sharing and implementation of best practices.

The following comprehensive lists of indicators have been developed by a number of obstetric units to try to identify triggers for review at regular audit and teaching meetings (these may be held weekly):

Obstetric indicators
Maternal death
Booked home delivery admitted to hospital
In utero transfer to another unit
Undiagnosed breech
Fetal trauma
Maternal convulsions/collapse
Failure to interpret or act on results/imaging
Difficult CTG interpretation
Refusal of consent
Drug error
Lack of facilities/drugs
Lack of appropriate supervision
Failed instrumental delivery
> 12 hours undelivered
> 90 minutes active pushing in second stage

Neonatal indicators
Unexpected stillbirth
Unexpected neonatal death
Apgar < 4 at 5 minutes
Difficult resuscitation
No paediatrician present at high-risk delivery
Birth trauma/injury
Meconium aspiration
Major congenital abnormality not detected
Unplanned admission to SCBU/NNU
Baby readmitted to SCBU/NNU
Seizure during first 3 days of life
Any paralysis
Subdural haematoma
Drug errors
Equipment failure

Obstetric indicators (*continued*)
> 30 minutes from decision to
incision for emergency LSCS
Emergency LSCS with poor outcome
Anaesthetic complications
Ruptured uterus
Unplanned return to theatre
Admission to ITU
Incorrect swab/instrument count
Equipment failure
Major obstetric haemorrhage
(> 1000 ml)
Blood transfusion
Shoulder dystocia
Serious soft tissue injury (e.g.
third-degree tear)
Unexpected fetal abnormality
Complications (e.g. DVT)
Postnatal re-admission

Effective indicator systems and near miss and clinical incident reporting can provide: essential information for education and development of staff; improvements in Trust documentation that can help to improve clinical practice; early identification of potential risk of clinical negligence cases, including the provision of details (such as statements from staff involved and their location); and an estimation of defensibility, liability and early settlement of potential or actual claims against the Trust. Incident reporting, complaints and claims management need to be brought together under one umbrella to allow effective information to inform the risk management processes and to allow them to become much more proactive, supporting the notion that prevention is better and cheaper than cure.

Clinical risk modification – the best methods of risk prevention

Communication with patients

Communication is the most powerful tool in clinical practice, and research has repeatedly shown that good communication skills result in better clinical outcomes, greater propensity to follow clinical recommendations, and reduced risk of clinical negligence and complaints (Wilson, 1999). Healthcare professionals must be aware of the stresses associated with illness and hospitalization, and must learn the importance of good listening and effective communication if they are to ensure high quality patient care. Good communication with the woman and her partner improves the quality of midwifery care and engenders trust in the midwife. In the review of legal cases discussed earlier in this chapter, there were very few complaints or claims from women or their partners who had discussed a clear plan of care and had had ongoing discussions with and trust in the midwife. Problems tended to arise when several midwives cared for a woman during her intrapartum care, where there were inconsistencies, failure to take notice of the woman's concerns or lack of involvement in the plan of care. Ninety-four per cent of problems in healthcare delivery are due to poor communication (Wilson, 1999).

The following checklist will help in avoiding some of the most common pitfalls:

- Listen carefully to what the woman says
- Make sure she understands what she is told
- Do not talk down to her or be condescending – take time to answer questions
- Identify any necessary facilities for non-English speakers – interpreters and advocacy workers should be available 24 hours a day
- Continuity of care and keeping the woman fully informed during the antenatal period will help to ensure that she understands the management of her pregnancy; she should be part of the decision-making process
- A courteous introduction and clear staff identification is essential
- Avoid inadvertent and unintentional communication
- Avoid frivolous or critical statements about colleagues
- Respect the patient's wishes, and avoid negative verbal and non-verbal cues
- Avoid jargon, terminology or any language that may not be understood by the woman or her partner.

There are three main qualities that are essential to good clinical practice and effective communication.

1. Integrity – the commitment to be honest and trustworthy in evaluating and demonstrating personal skills and abilities
2. Respect – the personal commitment to honour others' choices and rights in clinical care
3. Compassion – an appreciation that suffering and illness engender special needs for comfort and help.

Minimizing risk also requires practitioners to communicate effectively with one another (see Chapter 4). Members of the multidisciplinary team each have their own role, responsibilities and accountability, but all are closely related, and effective communication is essential to ensure safe and continuous care for mothers and babies.

In order to enhance teamworking and safe practice there must be an organizational structure with explicit audit criteria for monitoring and evaluation of lines of communication, supported by an external and internal communication strategy. The strategy is assisted by having a midwifery manager, sufficient supervisors of midwives, a designated senior midwife in charge of the delivery suite, a named midwife shift co-ordinator, and a clinical practice development midwife who has a leading role in teaching, advice and support for all other midwives. Each midwifery unit should also have a lead obstetrician and senior midwife who have responsibility for risk, quality and clinical governance.

Maintaining good practice with effective clinical teams

Teamwork is essential for good midwifery practice. It is an essential ingredient in establishing an open, trusting relationship with the patient, the patient's partner and family. Open communication between the patient and the midwife, as well as between the team members, is crucial in keeping the patient well informed of the pregnancy status. Often it is the disgruntled and dissatisfied patient who has been in conflict or disharmonious environments that pursues clinical negligence cases when there is an unexpected result.

It is important that all team members understand and appreciate the significance of their roles and responsibilities. The following criteria can be audited to ensure good quality standards of teamwork:

- Clear leadership with designated senior staff and succession planning for developing junior staff
- Clear values/standards that are measured, monitored and re-audited on a regular basis with practice and development changes
- Staff involvement in regular rostered multidisciplinary training sessions, audit and education sessions, e.g. 3-monthly CTG training and regular review of CTG tracings and difficult labours
- Communication and documentation of care
- Commitment to quality – staff should be able to demonstrate continuous quality improvements, undertake patient and staff satisfaction surveys regularly, and demonstrate an agenda for quality improvements from practices, complaints, near misses, incidents and indicators
- Clear organizational structure, chain of command and jump call policy, with regular drills, skills and contingency planning events to ensure effectiveness
- Full awareness of limits of competency, and an open, honest and participative culture to seek guidance, help and supervision
- Care for each member of the team by providing advice, support and ongoing performance review to ensure that the team members feel valued, motivated and an essential part of the team
- Clear guidelines/protocols and management plans that are monitored for compliance and are reviewed to ensure safe practices
- Clear criteria and patient management plans, especially for high-risk cases
- Sharing and passing on information within the team
- Open systems for juniors to seek help and opinions – a consultant present for at least 40 hours per week
- Good teamwork, and respect for all members of the clinical team and the women in their care.

Protocols, guidelines and multidisciplinary pathways of care

Any framework for clinical quality must be amenable to monitoring and assurance of compliance with the policies of the healthcare organization. An excellent way to achieve this is through multidisciplinary pathways of care (MPCs; Wilson, 1995) that have utilized clinical guidelines, standards, outcomes and variance analysis. MPCs can incorporate components of effective care, including evidence-based practice, clinical audit, change management, multidisciplinary working and performance management. 'Multidisciplinary' means that all members of the team should have an equal say, and although teams require a leader there is little doubt that effective teams allow individuals to take leadership for particular objectives or responsibilities of that team's performance. Effective teams who are self-managed, self-directed and accountable will identify problems with variations from their targets, and will have responsibility for correcting those problems for quality of care improvements. MPCs are being used in many midwifery units, using the multidisciplinary model to incorporate maternal input (including birth plans). They can minimize the clinical variations and ambiguity in care and thereby reduce exposure to risk. With good management and design they can improve the monitoring of outcomes, track deviations and variations in care, and replace most of the existing paperwork to provide true multidisciplinary documentation.

Documentation of midwifery care

The goals of risk prevention/modification in terms of documentation are:

1. To provide and document maximum quality of care
2. To recognize and clearly document events that may provide exposure to poor clinical care, poor outcomes, or complaints and litigation
3. To implement and record measures to reduce such exposure
4. To monitor and record outcomes to ensure quality of patient care.

The maintenance of clear, comprehensive and contemporaneous maternal and baby records is an essential part of good midwifery practice. Hand-held records are a means of sharing information and enhancing partnership with the woman, and are to be encouraged. Written records help to organize care across the team, and aim to ensure that deviations from normal are not missed and that any interventions are made appropriately. Cardiotocographs (CTGs) are a crucial part of the record and should be filed securely in a designated envelope or folder within the record. All traces should be clearly labelled with the mother's name, hospital number and date of birth, and should be dated and timed with all interventions written on the trace. All care management and care plans should be written on the tracing, even if it is to state 'wait and see'. All partograms and anaesthetic records should also be carefully stored. The records should be a complete, sequential, contemporaneous, legible and accurate record of care, with:

- Date, times and signatures/printed name on every entry
- Joint decisions and consent to treatment recorded
- All decisions recorded, even if this is to continue with the current management
- A record of any warning about risks of intervention
- A record of any refusal of treatment, together with any suggested alternatives and the decision taken with regard to these
- Abbreviations and shorthand kept to a minimum (or if possible avoided)
- The amount, consistency and presence of meconium in liquor noted
- A note of any complaints or concerns expressed by the mother
- CTGs, partograms and anaesthetic records carefully stored.

In addition to the efficient storage of clinical case notes, units must ensure that current protocols, transfer arrangements etc. are available to staff, and that when these are superseded by more up-to-date protocols, the old ones are archived. In a retrospective investigation, the policies in place at the relevant time will be examined to ascertain whether staff acted appropriately.

It is a good idea to review your patient-related documentation by asking:

1. Is it timely? Delays lead to sketchy records and inaccuracies.
2. It is objective? Describe events, but avoid frivolous statements and criticisms of care.
3. Are there any inappropriate terms, such as 'the baby was flat and blue'?
4. It is process orientated? Is the woman's response to interventions noted? Can the care be compared to your multidisciplinary standards and clinical risk standards?
5. Does it include reassuring information? This may be supported by reference to clinical guidelines, birth plans and patient information leaflets.
6. Is the entire record retrievable and legible? The idea of the record is to share the plan of care with all staff to enhance patient safety and quality of care.
7. Have any alterations been made? Remember that liquid paper should not be used.

Clinical governance

Under clinical governance there are certain requirements concerning documentation. These are essentially to ensure that the maximum amount of information is available when retrospective enquiries are necessary. Very often these relate to how well practitioners have identified and responded to risk factors – i.e. have staff carried out the necessary investigations, recognized higher levels of risk and involved the appropriate personnel?

There are various clinical outcomes that might be the subject of a review. Some are mandatory across the whole country (e.g. maternal deaths; stillbirths and deaths in infancy), while others may be determined by local audit (e.g. instances of *in utero* or neonatal transfer, other unplanned admission to a neonatal unit, or delay in Caesarean section).

Clinical audits of randomly selected records should take place on a regular and frequent basis. Supervisors of midwives have a responsibility to carry out audit to ensure that maternal records meet the required standards of practice. Many of the suggested aspects of good practice concerning documentation have already been mentioned. Quality assurance in this area may also include whether there is:

- Evidence of discharge instructions from the clinic, ward or department and the information provided to the woman
- Any evidence of documentation of patient teaching and preparation for theatre or procedures and family interaction
- Completed and consistent documentation of multidisciplinary care throughout the patient's full span of care within the maternity services
- Use of a signature bank to maintain a record of signatures and printed names.

The latter aspect is particularly important because many practitioners move from one hospital to another, some working for only a short time in one place. Retrospective identification may become extremely problematic.

The healthcare provider should be able to show demonstrable results in risk reduction from the clinical audit process. This should be developed by a multidisciplinary team, and should include (but not be limited to) the following:

- Clinically valid standards of care set by the team and incorporated into the maternal documentation, admissions via delivery suite, and the giving and recording of telephone advice
- Agreed standards of care set by the multidisciplinary team linked to multi-disciplinary pathways of care, protocols, policies and practice guidelines
- Midwifery supervisory monitoring of safe standards of practice
- Specific thresholds used to monitor compliance, with established standards, clinical guidelines and evidence-based practice
- Defined methods for the collection and analysis of data, including reference to collection tools, sample size, timeframe and staff responsibility
- Provisions for corrective action planning to include educational opportunities, organizational modifications and behavioural changes
- Evidence of follow-up assessment to evaluate the effectiveness of the corrective action and ongoing results and plans of care
- Recognition and maintenance of good practices.

Evaluation of patient care should include (but not be limited to) the following:

- Completeness and legibility of patient records, care plans, informed consent and investigation results
- Accuracy of diagnosis, interventions/procedures, treatment and follow-on care, including allergies and the care delivery processes
- Appropriateness of use of laboratory investigations, routine radiology procedures and other services
- The safe and secure movement of patients throughout the maternity services, and the recording and information communicated between staff
- The outcome of care in the short, medium and long term
- Review of patients who leave before examination and those who discharge against medical advice
- Reviews of patients with a mental health history and those intoxicated on arrival at the delivery suite.

Successful risk management is becoming less of a matter of procedures and more a matter of *teamwork* that manages the care and documents the processes appropriately, no matter where the healthcare delivery takes place. Working in teams also requires an effective two-way process of sharing of information and communication (see Chapter 4).

Security for staff, mothers and babies

The security of everyone within a maternity unit (and of clinical staff and patients in the community) is a major concern for employers. Assaults on healthcare practitioners have become more common (Elliott and Dvorak, 2000), and abductions of babies from maternity units, while thankfully rare, have also focused attention on the need to ensure that there is adequate security within units. A robust system includes:

- An effective system of staff identification
- Controlled access to wards and units

- One-worker policies for community midwives and staff working in isolation
- Strict criteria for labelling and security of the newborn infant
- Agreed criteria for home confinements.

Women's wishes and birth plans

Reasonable steps should be taken to comply with the woman's wishes and with her choices concerning antenatal, intrapartum and postnatal care. However, there may be occasions when, in the midwife's judgement, compliance with certain requests could conflict with acceptable practice and standards of care. Midwives are accountable practitioners – accountable not only to the women for whom they care, but also to their professional body and their employers. Midwives may at times encounter conflict when trying to balance all these factors (see, for example, Anderson, 1994). All steps should be clearly explained to the woman and her partner. Again it is with good communication and building up of trust and confidence that everyone understands and agrees with the plan of care. It is rare to see conflict in this area with independent midwifery or appropriately managed case midwifery where there is a true ongoing and good relationship with clients supported by excellent communication and decision-making.

Clinical risk modification – a midwifery improvement model

This model (Table 2.4) pulls together the basic principles of good clinical risk management. Appropriateness of care must be based upon having evidence-based research/practice to ensure that there are clear criteria on which to base best practice in order to have good reasoning as to why things should be done. These together will provide the best defense in terms of processes and systems if things do go wrong, and in having the quality assurance standards to demonstrate a controlled environment of care. This environment must be achieved in line with clinical and cost effectiveness to ensure that scarce resources are used to achieve the balance and not to practise defensive medicine for fear of litigation. The care provided can be demonstrated through the usage of multi-disciplinary pathway care, effective communication and good record keeping. Then it is possible to ensure the outcomes and identify whether practices work for the mother, her baby and her experiences of childbirth, as well as for clinical outcomes.

Table 2.4 Clinical risk modification – a midwifery improvement model

Appropriateness	Efficiency	Effectiveness
Clinical guidelines, reflective practice and integrated care	Multidisciplinary pathway care, communication and good record keeping	Clinical standards, supervision and outcome measurement
Should it be done?	How is it done?	Did it work?

Case study

The following case scenario highlights a number of risk issues that arose from failures to recognize the importance of teamworking and high-risk patients/ practices, and an inability to modify high-risk exposures. Not having models of midwifery improvements and ways of demonstrating appropriateness, clinical effectiveness and efficiency can result in unnecessary risk exposure through lack of recognition, poor teamworking, and the inability to apply ongoing risk assessments and modification of high-risk exposures.

The case illustrates the need for an effective planning process designed to support a collaborative approach to managing the care of high-risk patients. It emphasizes the benefits of pre-arranged agreements, integrated policies and procedures, and a well co-ordinated transfer process. The effective management of these shared patient care responsibilities can greatly enhance the quality of patient care and can minimize potential liability exposures for all providers and trusts involved.

Maternity care is usually uncomplicated and can be managed easily in a maternity unit in a general hospital. However, during pregnancy, complications may arise that require referral to a tertiary centre. Complicated or high-risk deliveries may necessitate maternal/fetal transfer or arrangements for the neonatal team to be present and to assume responsibility for neonatal care at the time of delivery. The care of some high-risk patients may involve a specialized regional centre, obstetric specialists, ambulance/helicopter transfer services, and neonatal intensive care unit (NICU) facilities.

The names and hospital details presented in the following case are fictitious in order to protect the individuals involved.

Mary Adams versus Rosehill Trust

Transfer: the importance of collaboration
Mary Adams arrived at Rosehill NHS Trust Hospital at 0200 hours on 7 February. She was obviously pregnant, and stated that her membranes had ruptured and she was having intermittent contractions. In addition, Ms Adams said she had received no antenatal care. Rosehill NHS Trust is a 300-bed hospital in a rural area of the country. The hospital is capable of providing basic obstetric care, but has no neonatal intensive care unit (NICU) or special care baby unit (SCBU).

On examination, Ms Adams was noted to be in established labour with her cervix 4 cm dilated and 90 per cent effaced. She was unsure of her gestation as she had a history of irregular periods. An ultrasound was performed, which revealed a twin pregnancy at an estimated 32-week gestation. The decision was made to transfer the patient immediately to a regional centre. Fetal heart rates were documented to be around 120 beats per minute.

A call was placed promptly to the University Trust Hospital Regional Centre to arrange the transfer. The patient's limited known history was relayed to the University Trust Hospital. Rosehill Trust was informed that the transfer could not take place as University Trust Hospital had no available beds. A second regional centre, Beechcroft NHS Trust, was then called. Beechcroft also refused to accept the transfer, as its transport team was currently unavailable.

Ms Adams' labour progressed rapidly. Twin boys were delivered at 0440 and 0442 hours. The first twin weighed 1420 g and had Apgar scores of 2 at 1 minute and 4 at 5 minutes; the second twin weighed 1360 g and had Apgar scores of 1 at 1 minute and 3 at 5 minutes. Both infants had difficulty establishing effective respirations. The midwifery staff performed bag and mask ventilation, but both babies required immediate intensive care. Ms Adams encountered no complications.

Immediately after delivery, another call was placed to a third Regional centre, the Royal Victoria NHS Trust, which accepted the transfer of the Adams twins. The Royal Victoria flying squad transport team arrived promptly, but received very little clinical information from Rosehill as the staff involved (there were only four members of staff on duty) were apparently called to attend another delivery. Both babies were intubated by the Royal Victoria flying squad staff and stabilized for transfer.

During the transfer to Royal Victoria, which was 40 miles away, both Adams twins began to have convulsions. Twin two died shortly after arrival at the Royal Victoria Trust. The first twin survived, but spent several months in the Royal Victoria Trust NICU. The baby was discharged with a questionable prognosis, to be followed in the developmental clinic. A subsequent examination at 9 months indicated that the surviving twin suffered from convulsions, cerebral palsy and significant developmental delay.

Allegations and claims issues
A clinical negligence claim was issued against Rosehill NHS Trust Hospital approximately 1 year after the delivery. Allegations included:

1. Failure to transfer Mary Adams to a Trust equipped to handle her delivery prior to the birth of her twin sons.

Rosehill NHS Trust Hospital had no written policies or protocols regarding the transfer of patients. There also were no transfer agreements with any Regional Centre Trusts. Several Rosehill staff nurses reported in their statements that similar transfers had been problematic in the past, particularly with patients who had undiagnosed multiple births or other complications.

2. Failure to call in the appropriate paediatric specialists to manage the care of the infants once delivery was imminent.

Rosehill had no written policies or protocols regarding the need for specialists, such as a neonatologist/paediatrician, to be present at delivery. In this case, a paediatrician was not present at the delivery and intubation was not requested or attempted.

3. Failure to have the appropriate hospital staff available to resuscitate the twin boys properly or to manage their care.

None of the midwives or doctors present at the delivery were trained/skilled in intubation or were able to intubate the babies. The plaintiff's expert witness testified that the complications encountered by both babies were the direct result of ineffective bag and mask resuscitation prior to the arrival of the Royal Victoria NHS Trust flying squad team.

4. Failure properly to transfer the infants, resulting in the death of one child and brain damage to the other twin.

The Rosehill NHS Trust medical record was completely absent of any documentation regarding the resuscitative efforts for the babies, other than a note that stated that the infants were being bagged and masked and that

Royal Victoria flying squad team were '*en route*'. The Royal Victoria medical record stated that the babies were accepted for transfer, but essentially no history or clinical information was received from the Rosehill NHS Trust.

This claim was ultimately settled prior to trial for a structured package costing in excess of £1 million.

The facts in the case illustrate significant responsibilities involved in patient transfers:

- Medical screening and stabilization prior to transfer
- Transfer agreements, policies and procedures
- Transition care prior to transfer.

Additional liabilities in the case related to inadequately trained staff, the failure to call in appropriate personnel (there was no available paediatrician/neonatologist), and failures in communicating appropriate medical information.

Patient transfers

Medical screening and stabilization

When delivery is imminent, there is inadequate time to effect a safe transfer to another hospital. Transfer may pose a threat to the health and safety of the woman or her unborn baby. This suggests that the responsibility for determining whether labour is advanced rests with the practitioners in the hospital. The hospital protocol should identify the staff responsible for such screening. Failure to have designated and available medical personnel can result in liability for the hospital.

While individual practitioners can be held negligent, an employing authority, in the way it organizes and delivers health care, can also be held liable (*cf.* Bull *v.* Devon HA [1993]). In this particular instance the failure to have a plan of management for such cases (including the failure to train staff in emergency procedures) may be seen as negligent.

Transfer plan

Once it was clear that the patient in the case was in active labour, the lack of an adequate transfer plan resulted in the inability to transfer the patient and led to a serious liability problem. As the 'Risk view' section below notes, pre-arranged policies and agreements should address the circumstances under which transfers will take place and provide guidance for all personnel involved in the transfer.

An integrated planning process can help small hospitals to demonstrate that reasonable efforts have been taken to support the safe transfer of patients who require services that they do not offer. Transfer planning must apply to all patients without regard to their NHS contract status or whether their GP is a fundholder.

Transition period prior to transfer

It is important to note that having protocols in place for transfer situations does not release the referring hospital from its legal responsibility to ensure that adequate care is rendered during any interim period between the initial medical evaluation and the actual time of transfer. Protocols that define the available medical coverage and the requirements for such coverage until the transfer also need to be in place.

If trained personnel from either Trust have not been designated to assume specific responsibilities during the transition period of care, legal liability could result.

The planning process includes consideration of:

- Procedures for identifying and managing patients requiring transfer (this includes having appropriately trained staff)
- Delineation of medical management responsibilities throughout the transfer process
- Co-ordination of protocols for maternal/neonatal transport and ambulance services
- The documentation of patient care activities and the sharing of patient care information/records
- Patient education and consent procedures
- Backup systems and alternative procedures for situations that may interfere with or delay needed transfers.

Risk view

Mary Adams was a high-risk obstetric patient when she presented to Rosehill NHS Trust Hospital with a history of no antenatal care, ruptured membranes and intermittent contractions at an unknown gestational age. Physical and ultrasound examinations confirmed active labour at 32 weeks with a twin pregnancy. Anticipation of a complicated delivery together with the potential need for neonatal intensive care services, not available at Rosehill, led to the appropriate decision to transfer Mary to a regional centre facility. The hospital's difficulty, however, in effecting a transfer as expeditiously as the clinical situation warranted, and the lack of a plan to address this problem, increased the patient's risk and created potential liability for the hospital.

The proactive development of a plan to support the appropriate transfer of high-risk patients who cannot be cared for safely within a NHS Trust is a critical element in ensuring patient safety and in reducing potential liability exposures. The fact that transfers had been problematic in the past should have spurred Rosehill to address this problem and enlist Regional centre staff to assist in the development of contingency plans. A comprehensive approach to planning for safe, effective transfers requires:

1. Clear recognition by the transferring Trust of its capabilities and limitations
2. Implementation of maternal–fetal/neonatal policies and procedures when tertiary beds are temporarily unavailable
3. Establishment of agreements between the referring and receiving Trusts regarding the acceptance of patients requiring transfer
4. Development and maintenance of a collaborative relationship with regional centres and neonatal intensive care units.

Recognition of capabilities and limitations

An in-depth review and clear delineation of the Trust's ability to provide care is crucial for the effective management of risk. This includes recognition of limitations, whether related to knowledge and skill of healthcare providers, equipment, staffing, geographic considerations, transport availability, anticipated response time, or other factors.

Once the hospital's capabilities and limitations are clearly recognized, criteria can be developed to identify those patients who should be considered for transfer to a Regional care centre. Formal development of such criteria, based on a realistic assessment of the Trust's capabilities, can be invaluable in identifying potential transfer candidates early and in guiding decision-making in difficult clinical situations.

Maternal–fetal/neonatal policies

Any Trust providing obstetric services must have personnel, equipment and systems capable of arranging timely emergency deliveries. This includes the resuscitation and stabilization of mothers and babies until care can be handed over to other providers. Written policies and protocols that delineate responsibility for providing safe care in the event that transfer is delayed need to be developed and approved by both the midwifery and medical staff. Identifying the need for initial and ongoing training and education and providing for regular updates and evaluation should be considered when developing policies and protocols.

In this case, Rosehill Trust failed to provide adequately for the resuscitation of the infants. The case implies that the bag and mask resuscitation procedure may not have been performed properly. This raises a question about the training and education of the midwifery and medical staff for this responsibility. In this case, where neonatal difficulties could and should have been anticipated, medical and midwifery personnel with documented training in infant resuscitation should have been available. It is essential in all high-risk deliveries to have appropriately trained practitioners present (usually a paediatrician/or neonatologist) to undertake resuscitation of newborn babies. These designated staff members should have been present in addition to the obstetrician, as well as competent personnel responsible for administering epidural anaesthesia (if required) to the mother.

Transfer agreements

Significant potential liability exposures exist for both referring hospitals (in releasing patients to the care of others) and regional centres (in sending flying squad personnel to transport high-risk patients). Activities and documentation in both Trusts should be guided by agreements and protocols established by the involved Trusts. The development of integrated procedures supporting safe, effective transfers should involve proactive input from multiple disciplines and departments from both Trusts, and may address such issues as:

- Access to antenatal care
- Identification of patients who are currently or are likely to become high risk

- Communication with and providing appropriate records to the hospital where delivery is expected to occur
- Which deliveries require a paediatrician or neonatologist to be present, especially if transfer arrangements are not possible
- Patient education about the hospital to which they should present themselves
- Responsibility for medical management during the transfer process
- Responsibility for documentation during the transition period
- Provision for evaluation of the transfer process by both Trusts.

Consensus should also be reached on procedures to be followed if the Trust Regional centre does not have a bed available or is unable to accept the transfer. Alternative transfer facilities and procedures may need to be designated.

Throughout the planning process, care should be taken to ensure that transfer policies are not dependent on contract status or the patient's Primary Care Trust. Inability to ensure that 'money follows the patient' should not be a risk factor in the decision-making process.

A collaborative relationship

An ongoing, collaborative relationship among Referral and Regional centres yields benefits to all. The Referral centres can benefit from increased avail ability of consulting services, heightened awareness of capabilities and limit-ations of both hospitals, and expanded opportunities for continuing education. Regional centres can benefit from opportunities to have a positive impact on the quality of prenatal network services, as well as the development of referral sources.

Good communication is vital to any collaborative transfer relationship. Fail-ure to provide an appropriate report and to document the findings, interventions and responses in adequate detail severely compromises the ability of a flying squad transport team to manage patient care and poses significant risk exposures to the Trust initiating the transfer.

The receiving hospital also has a responsibility to keep personnel from the referring hospital informed of the transferred patient's progress. Sending a copy of the discharge summary to the transferring obstetrician/paediatrician can provide important feedback to complete the loop. An effective communication system strengthens the connection between the referring and the receiving Trusts.

Conclusions

The goal of clinical risk modification is to improve the quality of midwifery care by improving the processes and systems of care and thereby reducing or minimizing the costs of failures. This chapter has covered much ground in terms of practical tips and experiences to allow readers to manage their risks more proactively. Further chapters in this book will go into some of the areas raised here in more depth, and will explore the practical application of clinical risk management. There are different ways of practising risk management, and thereby fully utilizing clinical risk modification; these usually start off in a reactive way (Table 2.5) and build up to being more proactive (Table 2.6) and preventative.

The potential benefits of a risk management programme should result in the features listed in Table 2.7.

The current stage of clinical risk management within an organisation should be easily identifiable, and the steps to be taken can be learned. One of the most important lessons that healthcare providers can learn is that risk management is a process, not a position. So often during reviews staff feel that because they

Table 2.5 Reactive risk management

- Learning lessons from things that have gone wrong and from near misses and cases selected from clinical indicators
- Correction of errors and trying to ensure they do not happen again
- Analysis of complaints, near misses, incidents and claims, with tracking, trending and sharing of information and implementation of practice changes and lessons learned
- Management of complaints, near misses, incidents and claims in a proactive way rather than being defensive and personalizing the issues being raised
- Minimization of distress and providing support to staff and clients
- Management of claims including clinical involvement
- Risk containment
- Risk control

Table 2.6 Proactive risk management

- Identification of existing risk, ensuring risk awareness and controls are in place and are used in everyday practice
- Assessment of potential systems failure and having contingency/disaster plans and drills and skills training to practise for all eventualities
- Analysis of priorities for action, ensuring there is ongoing review and prioritization of risks
- Changes in practices, behaviour and culture of the organization supported by good change management and organizational development techniques
- Elimination/reduction of hazards to ensure risks are controlled, transferred or managed, and making staff aware of the changes with re-audit to test for the levels of effectiveness
- Incorporating quality, risk and audit into one department of clinical effectiveness, led by the midwifery team, and part of the agenda of ongoing weekly meetings
- Use of integrated care management and multidisciplinary pathways of care in working in partnership with colleagues, mothers and their partners for seamless, high-quality care, demonstrated by standards and outcome measures
- Addressing clinical effectiveness and patient outcomes to ensure appropriateness of care through clinical and cost effectiveness, evidence-based practice and research.

Table 2.7 Potential benefits of clinical risk management

- Improvements in quality of care
- Reduction in damage and injury to mothers and babies
- A safer environment for the provision of midwifery services
- Increased wellbeing of staff, and good teamworking
- Full utilization of audit and perinatal meetings, including case review, indicator, near miss and incident reporting
- Management of future uncertainty with better predictability and care management with optimal maternity outcomes
- Cost and clinical improvement benefits
- Meeting the requirements of corporate and clinical governance and being able to demonstrate clear accountability, controls and maternal outcomes.

have a risk manager, that person has responsibility and accountability for risk; in fact risk management is and should be part of everyone's role and responsibility and should be an element of job plans and individual objectives of all midwives. In order to meet the quality focus of the NHS, clinical risk modification must be achieved through safe and effective practices.

References

Anderson, T. (1994). Trust betrayed: the disciplining of the East Herts midwives. *MIDIRS Midwifery Digest*, **4(2)**, 132–4.

Department of Health (1997). *The New NHS: Modern, Dependable*. HMSO Cmnd 3807.

Elliott, P. P. and Dvorak, M. A. (2000). Preventing violence in the health care setting. *Mother Baby J.*, **5(3)**, 23–8.

Law, D., Lewington, T., Fletcher, R. and Hawkins, C. (1996). Allegations of medical negligence against hospitals in the West Midlands region. *J. MDU*, **12(3)**, 67–9.

Maternal and Child Health Research Consortium (1998). *Confidential Enquiry into Stillbirths and Deaths in Infancy*, 7th Report. MCHRC.

Maternal and Child Health Research Consortium (2000). *Confidential Enquiry into Stillbirths and Deaths in Infancy*, 7th Report. MCHRC.

Sanderson, I. M. (1998). The CNST: a review of its present function. *Clinical Risk*, **4**, 35–42.

Wilson, J. (1995). Risk focus: a collaborative approach to perinatal transfers. *Health Care Risk Report*, **April**.

Wilson, J. (1996). *Integrated Care Management: The Path to Success*. Butterworth-Heinemann.

Wilson, J. (1999). In: *Clinical Risk Modification: A Route to Clinical Governance* (J. Wilson and J. Tingle, eds), Butterworth-Heinemann.

Law Case:

Bull *v.* Devon HA [1993] 4 Medical Law Reports 117.

3

The midwife and the legal environment

Andrew Symon

Introduction

Why have legal issues become such a fixation within health care? The plethora of study days for healthcare workers – especially midwives and obstetricians – are an indication that there is considerable concern within the health service about the threat of litigation. There is no doubt, too, that a certain amount of publicity in the general media highlights the possibility of legal recourse when an outcome is suboptimal. Lastly, users of the health service have been informed that it is their right to complain if certain standards are not met, and some of these complaints come in legal form.

This chapter is divided into three parts. The first notes apparent changes in lay perceptions and expectations that are assumed to have fuelled the increase in complaints and litigation, and places obstetrics/midwifery in perspective from the limited data published by the medical defence organizations. The second gives an account of the civil law relating to clinical negligence, discusses possible developments within this, and notes the principal allegations of negligence levied against practitioners involved in perinatal care. The third concerns risk management, and explores the clinical implications of litigation based on features noted in the literature and in personal research, illustrating this with examples from actual cases.

Lay expectations

'Blessed is the man who expects nothing, for he shall never be disappointed' was the ninth beatitude.

(Alexander Pope, 1725)

Expectations and perceptions

Although this book concerns midwifery, and raises the question of societal expectations with regard to pregnancy and childbirth, it is fair to acknowledge that the public's expectations, and raised expectations in particular, are a concern for many different professional and organizational groups. A brief search of the literature confirms that the place of expectations concerns those in areas as diverse as higher education (Shank and Hayes, 1995), social work training (Kerson, 1994), tourism (Dann, 1996) and restaurants (Clow *et al.*, 1996), to name just a few. Nevertheless, the presence of raised expectations within maternity care poses certain distinct challenges for those who organize and provide the service (Symon, 2001).

There is a considerable literature regarding the expectations and experiences of those who use the maternity services (e.g. O'Meara, 1993; Avis *et al.*, 1997). Antenatal teaching/parenthood education has seen the development of birth plans in recent years as a means of trying to inform the pregnant woman about possible choices, particularly with reference to her labour. Beaton and Gupton (1990) note that: 'inherent in the development of birth plans is the danger that women may be encouraged to think that planning the "perfect" birth is possible'. Are midwives, without realizing it, suggesting that there is a right not only to a personally fulfilling experience, but also to a perfect baby?

While it is easy to criticize this view, it is clear that some practitioners do believe that health professionals have, albeit inadvertently, contributed to expectations that are sometimes unrealistic (Symon, 1998a, 1998b). Bastian (1990) claims that obstetricians have 'deliberately or not, fostered a consumer perception that, essentially, childbirth can be more or less controlled and babies can be saved if only enough money is spent on the appropriate technology'. Ellis (1988, p. 9) similarly notes that, birth plans aside, 'a vastly inflated concept of medicine's capacity to overcome all the ills of mankind leads quite a number of people to interpret the right to health care as a right to health'.

When such expectations are not met, there is the possibility of a complaint (the Patient's Charter and other similar local initiatives advertise this) or even a formal allegation of negligence. However, it is important not to overstate this possibility: certain studies have tried to indicate why people do sue (Vincent *et al.*, 1994), while other reports have indicated a reluctance to pursue this line despite encouragement (Lindsay, 1994). In explaining why some don't sue (although grounds for doing so may exist), Lamont (1993) cites deference and a fear of taking on the establishment.

It may be tempting to assume that midwifery and obstetrics have been singled out as a particular target for litigants, but there are claims that many different areas have experienced an increase in complaints and litigation. Dingwall (1994) notes that architects, accountants, veterinary surgeons, engineers and even lawyers have encountered increasing levels of litigation. Nevertheless, it does appear that when the person allegedly harmed is a baby or a newly-delivered mother, the subject is particularly newsworthy.

The emotiveness of the baby image is particularly striking: advertisers have seen the potential appeal of the baby, and used newborn infants to sell products from nappies and washing powder (fairly obvious) to motor cars, and private health insurance, and even to promote a supermarket chain (a less clear-cut connection). The overused image of a happy smiling baby may be held to contribute to the expectation that every pregnancy will result in such a blissful outcome. With reference to notions of replacing sanctity of life issues with quality of life issues, Diamond (1980, p. 133) notes this 'cult of perfection', and criticizes the current view that 'Vita is not vita unless it is La Dolce Vita'. This subject is covered further in Chapter 6.

The effect on the health service

We must conclude that, in general, people today are less prepared to accept what they perceive to be an unsatisfactory outcome. Within the health service, avenues for pursuing complaints have been made widely known, and the possibility of legal redress for perinatal incidents has received publicity in the general media (e.g. Anon, 1997a; McKain, 2000; Fresco, 2000). The medical press have not been slow to identify litigation as a significant factor (e.g. Black, 1990; Saunders, 1992; Tharmaratnam and Gillmer, 1995), and the midwifery and nursing press have followed suit (Acheson, 1991; Anon, 1997b). Legal journals, unsurprisingly, have long been discussing this matter (Howie, 1983; Easterbrook, 1996), and sadly there is no shortage of recently reported legal cases concerning midwives (e.g. Wisniewski *v.* Central Manchester HA [1996]; Corley *v.* NW Hertfordshire HA [1997]; Gaughan *v.* Bedfordshire HA [1997]).

Medical Protection Society (MPS) figures released in the late 1980s acknowledged that while those involved in obstetrics and gynaecology made up 3 per cent of their membership at that time, they accounted for 29 per cent of claims made and 36 per cent of the amount paid out in damages (MPS, 1989). Subscription levels for all the Medical Defence Organizations (MDOs) rose sharply in the 1980s (Ham *et al.*, 1988), and then fell with the introduction of NHS indemnity for hospital doctors in 1990. Since then, however, the perceived threat of litigation has caused MPS rates to rise again sharply, particularly for those practising obstetrics outwith the NHS; in 1992 a special new category, 'obstetric risk', was introduced for which premiums are higher than for all the other specialties considered 'high risk'.

This perceived threat for those involved in perinatal care has also spread to independent midwives in Britain. For years covered by the indemnity insurance automatically conferred by membership of the Royal College of Midwives (RCM), in 1994 they were perceived by the RCM's insurer as carrying too high a risk, and cover for this small group of practitioners was withdrawn.

Expectations, it seems, have increased. With this, practitioners, and especially those involved in maternity care, have found themselves increasingly the subject of complaints (Warden, 1996) and legal claims. The next section details how the civil law operates in this area.

Clinical negligence and the midwife

Introduction

The law operates in a number of different ways, each of which can affect the perinatal practitioner. There is of course the criminal law; a celebrated case in 1925 saw an obstetrician both sued in the civil courts and prosecuted in the criminal courts for his conduct at a delivery. More recently, Henderson (1997) reports that an obstetrician faces manslaughter charges 'after a coroner halted an inquest ... and referred papers about the death of a newborn baby to the Crown Prosecution Service'. Thankfully this side of the law rarely applies to clinical practitioners, as conduct has to be criminally negligent to involve prosecution by the state.

While the criminal law acts by punishing, the civil law – with which we are concerned here – attempts to compensate someone who has suffered loss or damage through negligence. The civil law, of course, covers many different areas that may affect the practitioner – employment, contractual and personal injury law being examples. This chapter is concerned with a form of personal injury law that has received a good deal of publicity in recent years, namely clinical negligence. This covers all clinical practitioners involved in the delivery of health care, and so covers midwifery. Personal injury litigation is covered by the law of torts (wrongs); this is called delict in Scotland.

There is a theory of deterrence in a tort/delict system (i.e. the fear of litigation encouraging safe practice), and this may be seen as proactive. However, the civil law in this field is essentially reactive: personal injury law acts retrospectively to put someone in the position he or she would have been in had the untoward event/accident not happened. This means that the law is restitutive in nature: it aims to restore the *status quo ante*. The law cannot of course cure a cerebral palsy, heal a damaged perineum or restore a dead child to life. All it is in a position to do is to improve a situation through financial compensation. This is an important point to note when considering whether anyone has the right to a perfect baby, for the law cannot ensure this. All it can do in the event of a poor outcome caused by negligence is to try to ameliorate that bad position through compensation.

This chapter, then, approaches the question of a practitioner's contact with the law in terms of a particular aspect of the civil law, and specifically in terms of a particular type of personal injury litigation. There have been developments in the way the civil law is applied in this field, and these are covered towards the end of Chapter 10 in the section 'The new civil procedure rules and the pre-action protocol'.

Clinical negligence

To establish clinical negligence (which used to be termed 'medical negligence'), the claimant must show that the defendant owed a duty of care; that there was a breach of this duty of care; and that damage resulted from the breach. The 'duty of care' principle stems from the judgement given in the case of Donoghue *v.* Stevenson [1932], and is sometimes referred to as the 'good neighbour' principle. In discussions relating to health care, it can be assumed that a practitioner (e.g. midwife, nurse or doctor) owes a duty of care to a patient.

There is a slight distinction between Scotland and England in terms of the law of clinical negligence. The test in Scotland was laid down in the judgement of Lord President Clyde in Hunter *v.* Hanley in 1955:

> *The true test for establishing negligence on the part of a doctor is whether he has been proven to be guilty of such failure as no doctor of ordinary skill would be guilty of if acting with ordinary care ... it must be established that the course the doctor adopted is one which no professional man of ordinary skill would have taken if he had been acting with ordinary care.*

This position was reaffirmed in the (English) case of Maynard *v.* West Midlands RHA in 1984, when the House of Lords held that in medicine there is room for a difference of opinion and practice, and that a court's preference for one body of opinion over another is no basis for a conclusion of negligence.

Hunter *v.* Hanley 1955 was followed 2 years later in English law in the case of Bolam *v* Friern HMC, and it is this case to which most legal texts refer. Lord McNair stated that:

> ... *the test as to whether there has been negligence or not is ... the standard of the ordinary skilled man exercising or professing to have that special skill ... He is not guilty of negligence if he has acted with a practice accepted as proper by a responsible body of medical men skilled in that particular art.*

One jurist notes that the Scottish and English tests for establishing an acceptable standard are slightly different: Howie (1983) claims that in Scotland the test for negligence (*per* Hunter *v.* Hanley 1955) is that no doctor of ordinary skill would have acted in the way alleged. In England, the Bolam principle holds that the act is safe as long as it is in accordance with a responsible body of opinion. In other words, he is claiming that the test in Scotland is tougher than in England. Another (anonymous) writer echoes this point, noting that in Maynard *v.* West Midlands RHA [1984] Lord Scarman said 'I do not think that the words of Lord President Clyde in Hunter *v.* Hanley can be bettered', but in the later case of Sidaway *v.* Board of Governors of the Bethlem Royal Hospital and others [1984] he referred to Bolam in detail and tried to equate Scots law with Bolam principles (Anon, 1990). As the two are not exactly the same, this commentator claims that the law in England is 'in an unsatisfactorily fluid state'. It must be said that this distinction is not a problem that seems to have troubled most writers or judges since the two respective judgements. The applicability of the Bolam test has recently been criticized in England (see below).

Liability cannot be inferred simply because something goes wrong. Lord Ross gave express approval of this in 1981 in the case of Rolland *v.* Lothian Health Board 1981:

> *If medical and nursing staff were to be found liable when anything untoward occurred, that would have an adverse effect on the medical and nursing professions and on the public generally.*

Brazier (1987, p. 76) picks up on this point of muzzling innovation:

> *If liability in negligence automatically followed once harm resulted from the adoption of a novel method of treatment, medical progress would be stultified.*

Causation

To establish negligence, a direct causal link between the breach of a duty and ensuing damage must be established. It is usually obvious in the case of a healthcare professional and a patient that there is a duty of care owed; it may also be evident that damage has been caused, but the causal link may be challenged. In Barnett *v.* Chelsea HMC [1968] it was established that a man had died after inadvertently drinking from a cup that had contained arsenic. Although he had presented at hospital with abdominal pains, he was not examined by the doctor but told to go and see his own GP. The duty of care owed had been breached – as the man had died it was obvious that harm had somehow been caused – but it was also established that the man would have died in any case because nothing the Casualty Officer might have done would have made any difference, and so there was no causal link.

The role of the experts

A legal dispute will often turn to the question of what should have happened in a particular case in order to see whether there might have been a breach of the duty of care. 'Expert opinions' may be sought to find out what the ordinary competent practitioner could be expected to do or know, and one of the hallmarks of a profession is that it reserves the right to decide just what is acceptable. This is noted by Klein (1973, p. 3): 'It is for professional colleagues, not the user of the services, to judge the appropriateness and the competence of the skills applied'. This view does not go unchallenged, however: Norrie (1985, p. 137) claims that medicine should be just as accountable as other occupations – 'It is nothing short of dangerous complacency to assume that they (doctors) are safe from legal criticism if they do only as their neighbours do'.

This view seemed to be backed up by the judgement given in the Court of Appeal case of Sidaway: 'the definition of a duty of care is a matter for the law and the court ... in a word, the law will not permit the medical profession to play God' (Lord Donaldson in Sidaway *v.* Bethlem Royal Hospital [1984]). A statement like this from such a senior judge usually carries great weight, and yet courts appear to have been happy to accept – within the bounds of reason-ableness – that in medical matters medical people are best placed to decide what is a satisfactory standard of care. A problem does however occur when 'expert witnesses' disagree with one another. In Whitehouse *v.* Jordan and another [1981] it was stated that 'expert opinion' must be seen to be the independent expert opinion of a specialist, and not partisan (*per* Lord Wilberforce, cited by Hodgson, 1981):

> *While some degree of consultation between experts and legal advisers is entirely proper, it is necessary that expert evidence presented to the court should be, and should be seen to be, the independent product of the expert uninfluenced as to form or content by the exigencies of litigation. To the extent that it is not, the evidence is likely to be not only incorrect, but also self-defeating.*

This view was reinforced by Thomas J in Wisniewski *v.* Central Manchester HA [1996]. With reference to one of the defence experts he said:

> *Professor Thomas' unwillingness to criticize was in my view unjustified and an example of his general disinclination to say much that might be adverse to the defendant's case.*

The importance of understanding the role of the expert is stressed in the training given by the Expert Witness Institute and the Judicial Committee of the Academy of Experts, which are both based in London. There is also advice for midwives and doctors on how to prepare for such a role (Copperfield, 1996; Dimond, 1996), and lists of suitable experts are held by the Royal Colleges (the Law Society also maintains the Expert Witness Register).

The test for clinical negligence, then, is that there is such a low standard of care given by a healthcare professional to someone to whom a duty of care is owed, that no practitioner of reasonably competent ability could have given that care, and that damage results from this. Given that the professions themselves are able to determine what is a reasonable standard of care, the test might appear to be a very tough one. This may be seen as one of the benefits accruing to a profession – that it has a strong say in how it will be judged by the law.

Criticisms of the law

The law of clinical negligence has been criticized in a number of different ways, and several options for reform have been suggested. These are briefly spelt out in this and the following section.

One criticism concerns the supposed effectiveness of deterrence in a tort/ delict system. Some argue that a free market contractual approach would enhance the deterrence of future mistakes, with a patient entering into negotiations with a doctor over the matter of liability. Others claim that the tort/delict system neither provides an adequate guarantee of compensation for those wronged, nor deters poor clinical standards, and so advocate a combination of increased regulation and no-fault compensation. Still others claim that the problem is due to a high propensity to sue, and so believe that doctors should be protected by restricting patient access to the courts (*cf.* Dingwall *et al.*, 1991).

The fact that a profession can determine what is a 'reasonable standard' has also been criticized in recent years. The Bolam approach is sometimes characterized unflatteringly as 'The doctor's friend', the argument being that if a healthcare professional can find colleagues who are deemed to be responsible to say that they would have acted in the same way, then negligence cannot be established. This is not in fact true, as was demonstrated in the recent case of Dowdie *v.* Camberwell HA [1997], which concerned a baby born with an Erb's palsy. Maurice Kay J stated:

> *The mere fact that two distinguished expert witnesses have testified that it was within the range of acceptable practice to proceed in that way does not oblige me to accept their evidence, and on this issue I accept the evidence of the plaintiff's experts.*

The debate about this reached some prominence in 1993: in Bolitho *v.* City & Hackney HA [1993] in the Court of Appeal Dillon LJ said:

> *In my judgement, the court could only ... reject medical opinion on the ground that the reasons of one group of doctors do not really stand up to analysis, if the court, fully aware of its own lack of medical knowledge and clinical experience, was nonetheless clearly satisfied that the views of that group of doctors were ... views such as no reasonable body of doctors could have held.*

However, the dissenting judge in this case (Simon Brown J) distinguished between applying the Bolam principle to the standard of care criterion and applying it to the question of causation, around which Bolitho turned:

> *The test outlined in Bolam and Maynard arose specifically in the context of negligence, and its use as the test of causation is inappropriate. The correct approach is rather to require the plaintiff to establish that the defendant's negligence materially contributed to his injury, which requires the court to consider what probably would have occurred had the doctor not been negligent ...*

This approach would give considerable leeway to the courts to disregard the evidence brought on behalf of a defendant, and is a prospect that some lawyers clearly relish. Goldrein (1994) claims it is surprising that the courts have allowed the medical profession to retain this sovereignty over evidence when they (the courts) have jealously asserted their rights to determine such matters in other fields. Another suggestion has been to shift the balance of proof concerning causation from the plaintiff to the defendant (Foster, 1996), which again erodes the position of the health professional.

The Bolitho case subsequently went to the House of Lords, and although the claim still did not succeed, the 'Bolam test' appeared to be qualified to the extent that 'the court had to be satisfied that the exponents of the body of opinion relied upon could demonstrate that such an opinion had a logical basis' (cited by Scott, 1998). This is in effect a 'reasonableness test': practitioners must satisfy a non-medical person (the judge) that the course of action was logical. As such, the right of doctors and midwives to determine what a reasonably competent practitioner ought to do or know is qualified. This may make defending allegations of negligence much harder.

Organizational alternatives

Leaving aside possible changes to the law of clinical negligence itself, several organizational alternatives have been advocated. These include appeals for more openness on the part of the health service, particularly with regard to giving explanations and apologies and allowing access to case notes (Beech, 1990); procedural changes to speed up the assessment of each case (Clothier, 1989); changes in the way Trusts deal with the financial side of litigation (Fenn and Dingwall, 1995; Easterbrook, 1996); attempts to encourage arbitration or mediation as an alternative to formal litigation (DoH, 1991; Dyer, 1995); and calls for no-fault compensation to be introduced (Ham *et al.*, 1988; Dyer, 1990).

A committee chaired by Lord Woolf, set up to find ways of improving access to civil justice in England and Wales, strongly backed the use of mediation in its interim report (Woolf, 1996). Now commonly used in divorce cases as well as small-scale disputes (such as those between neighbours), it is hoped that this will avoid the adversarial nature of the tort/delict system. A pilot study co-ordinated by the Oxford Centre for Medical Risk Studies, and funded by a number of hospital Trusts, aims to introduce mediation into medical accident or negligence cases, with a neutral third party acting as a go-between. Backing this move, Desmond, secretary of the Personal Injury Lawyers Group, claimed: 'The whole thing creates tremendous potential for settling clinical negligence claims before they get priced out of all sense of reality' (cited in Dyer, 1995). Genn (1999) notes that people who opt for mediation do so in order to avoid confrontation, and in the hope that settling the dispute will be less expensive and less time-consuming.

Those involved in maternity care (as in every other area of health care) are subject to the law, both criminal and civil. While criminal prosecutions are extremely rare, the civil law is a busy field. Some of the features of the law, in particular alternative methods of dispute resolution, may be set to change. However, as the law stands, a practitioner may be accused of negligence and all midwives must know how the law may affect them. The following section charts the allegations that have been made concerning perinatal care.

Experience of the law

Litigation in perinatal care, like risk management, is a multidisciplinary phenomenon. Because the care given to pregnant women and their babies comes from a range of disciplines, it is often not possible to distinguish the experience of different groups of practitioners. A woman making an allegation of negligence may have received care from a midwife, an obstetrician and an anaesthetist during her labour, and may also come into contact with paediatric and other neonatal staff while in hospital. Because of the complexity of these issues, and because some legal claims straddle the labour and neonatal periods, the following analysis of legal claims makes no distinction between the practitioners involved.

Types of claim

The debate about litigation in obstetrics/midwifery has focused largely on the issue of cerebral palsy. Such cases are deemed to be newsworthy: they involve a handicapped baby or child, a distressed family, and the possibility of hundreds of thousands or even millions of pounds in compensation. However, the reality is rather more complicated than this: Figure 3.1 shows the allegations made in over 600 perinatal legal cases (mostly originating in Scotland, but with over 100 from England) between 1980 and 1996. It shows how many cases are still ongoing, and the result of closed cases.

It is important to note that these are the allegations that have been made, and that the existence of an allegation does not necessarily indicate that negligence has occurred. Indeed, Figure 3.1 shows that the success rate for claimants is low, at around 28 per cent overall and only 27 per cent for the cases involving CNS

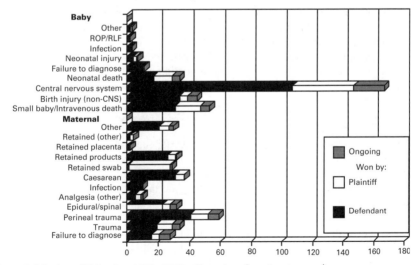

Figure 3.1 Perinatal litigation 1980–1996: allegations* and outcomes‡.
*Abbreviations: CNS, Central nervous system; ROP, Retinopathy of prematurity; RLF, Retrolental fibroplasia.
‡Outcome of claims for non-CNS (March 1999) and for CNS (March 2000). Earlier analysis of these claims, see Symon (1999). Reprinted with permission.

damage in the baby. However, the low success rate (compared with other personal injury litigation), while perhaps a matter of relief for practitioners, masks the emotional trauma involved.

In attempting to compare the experience of midwives and obstetricians – and related research suggests that obstetricians are far more likely to have been involved in litigation (Symon, 1998b) – there is a complicating factor. Because pregnant women have traditionally booked under the care of a consultant obstetrician, that consultant has in the past been named in legal actions even when the allegation of negligence concerns only midwifery or other non-medical (such as laboratory) staff. While this has skewed the rate of involvement towards obstetricians, this may be about to change with the continued development of the 'named midwife' concept and the growth of midwife-only care. Although the prospect of increased involvement in litigation is something that hardly appeals, it is the inevitable corollary of increasing autonomy (and accountability) for the midwife.

The important fact to highlight in this section is that allegations of negligence cover many different clinical areas. While the majority concern the intrapartum period, this area is complex, and there are also many cases from the antenatal and postnatal periods. The following section explores some of the clinical implications of such allegations.

Clinical implications

The involvement of midwives/obstetricians in clinically based litigation covers a number of areas, as was shown in Figure 3.1. While at first glance this seems to indicate a whole series of possible implications for clinical practice, in fact the features that are most heavily implicated in the origin of legal cases are relatively few, and are already by and large well known. Several reports and studies that have examined poor outcomes and litigation (e.g. James, 1991; Vincent *et al.*, 1991; MCHRC, 1997) have identified issues that were much in evidence in the examination of legal files referred to here. The principal themes are supervision, documentation, communication and use of the CTG, and in one way or another are all addressed by the concept of risk management.

Risk management

Risk management covers many different areas, including clinical competence, and the health and safety of all who enter a hospital (see Chapter 8). Even within maternity care it seeks to address a number of issues in an attempt to minimize the incidence of poor outcomes. While it certainly aims to reduce potential exposure to litigation, it should not be concluded that risk management is only concerned with minimizing expenditure on legal claims, although this is now a serious consideration for health service managers.

Several topics are discussed in this section. While many of these topics may seem obvious, if the problems caused by failing to implement the suggestions made were rare, they would not be cited here (*cf.* Cohn, 1984). In order to ground the discussion in a way that practitioners will find familiar, brief extracts are given from some of the legal cases that have been personally examined by the author.

Clinical risk management aims to minimize the incidence of adverse out-comes, and to facilitate effective claims management by establishing early client contact and ensuring that all relevant documents are completed (Dineen, 1996). Within obstetrics and midwifery – and in terms of risk management (as well as litigation) it must be conceded that perinatal care is a multidisciplinary field – there are several areas that can be targeted. In this discussion, risk and claims management are considered together. Claims management – the sensitive handling of claims when they come in – is in effect a sub-set of risk manage-ment, since its aim is still to minimize the risk of a damaging outcome.

Training and supervision

Inadequate supervision, both of patients and of junior staff, has been cited as a feature of perinatal legal actions (Ennis and Vincent, 1990; Doherty and James, 1994), and may relate to both midwives and obstetricians. Employers have a duty to ensure that junior staff are sufficiently supervised until their competence is assured. Competence cannot be assumed simply because a practitioner has been in post for a few weeks or even months. In this regard locum or agency staff present a particular problem; although qualified, their competence and skill may not have been demonstrated in that particular unit. Beard and O'Connor (1995) recommend that full supervision by a member of the regular staff be carried out. For medical staff, this may be effected by introducing dedicated consultant sessions in the labour ward – a move supported by the Royal College of Obstetricians and Gynaecologists (RCOG).

It is also the case that in many maternity units, relatively junior medical staff require to be supervised by midwives. An example of a failure to do this is given:

> *Without consulting a more senior colleague a Senior House Officer decided to use oxytocic drugs to augment a labour, when there was already evidence of fetal compromise. The woman had had a Caesarean section and cervical cryosurgery in the past, and had an epidural in situ. The uterus ruptured vertically through the cervix.*

Unsurprisingly, this case was settled by the defence. The question of supervision may be viewed in a number of lights: it may be argued that the SHO ought to have contacted a more senior colleague before taking this course of action, or that, alternatively, the relevant registrar ought to have been keeping a closer eye on this junior member of staff. Protocols establishing a need to inform a senior obstetrician when such procedures are contemplated may help. However, criticism may also be levelled at the midwifery staff who presumably did not challenge this course of action or demand that a more senior obstetrician attend. Effective communication with colleagues requires mutual respect. It is disheart-ening to note, therefore, that the standard of communication and rapport between midwife and doctor is widely believed to deteriorate significantly when a clinical situation worsens (Symon, 1998b). Risk management needs to address such inter-professional relationships, for without a shared view of the common aim of maternity care, suboptimal outcomes are much more likely. This is discussed in Chapter 4.

Communication

Poor communication has been highlighted as a factor in suboptimal outcomes (Dillner, 1995). Communication must be effective not only between practitioners and the women under their care, but also between different staff members. Drife (1995, p. 139) calls for a 'clear definition of the [midwife's] role vis-à-vis SHOs'. If midwives believe that a woman's pregnancy or labour has crossed the boundary from normal to abnormal, but cannot (for whatever reason) communicate this to the medical staff, then there is a problem. Drife (1995, p. 134) acknowledges that the hierarchy within a hospital can cause difficulties: 'A midwife may be frustrated by a doctor who does not respond appropriately to her concerns: yet she may be reluctant to "go over the head" of a junior doctor to a more senior doctor'.

Beard and O'Connor (1995) also note that the sharing of care between doctor and midwife can be problematic: 'Experience has shown that risk is increased if a midwife retains care for too long, or if a doctor, out of ignorance or faulty decision making, fails to accept responsibility for such a case'. In a situation like this it is imperative that practitioners communicate effectively. Good relationships may be helped through setting up an informal forum for the discussion of particular cases. Such an initiative must at all costs avoid becoming a 'finger-pointing' exercise, since that would destroy any hope of the mutual respect that underpins effective communication.

Communication between staff and the labouring woman and (where appropriate) her family is vital too. The following legal case concerned a family whose child developed cerebral palsy, with the mother claiming additionally for the pain and suffering she allegedly suffered at the time of her Caesarean section. The expert report stated:

> There has been no medical mismanagement ... {but} throughout the entire time there has been poor and unsympathetic communication with this unfortunate lady and while this cannot be quantitated in a legal sense it has been the major cause of her grievance.

In another case a couple went to see staff to seek an explanation of events, but subsequently sued because they felt 'angry at the flippant manner in which the case was treated'. Effective claims management begins before the notification of complaint or claim. In the event of any poor outcome or perceived grievance, practitioners are required to ensure that the woman and her family are kept informed, and that their questions are dealt with honestly and sensitively. Failing to do this will certainly increase the likelihood of a formal complaint or even a legal claim. The fact that there has indeed been no clinical negligence (as in the case cited above) will not stop this happening.

The overlap between obstetrics and neonatology can also provide room for communication-based mistakes to be made, or simply for women and their families to receive conflicting opinions. In one case a consultant neonatologist noted that:

> Difficulties of communication were compounded by threats of legal action against the obstetricians during the phase of critical illness of this infant.

In another case a baby was readmitted at 8 days of age with a history of seizures. When the paediatrician found no obvious cause for this, he apparently told the parents the condition was birth-related. However, with hindsight he acknowledged that the boy's problems were 'more severe than can be easily explained on the basis of the forceps delivery'. There is little doubt that his original assertion fuelled the legal claim, and the expert report criticized his injudicious expression of an opinion.

In maternity care we are often dealing with extreme emotions. When an outcome is poor, the suffering and distress experienced by all those involved can inhibit good communication. Staff may feel threatened in such an event, but whatever anguish practitioners may feel will not compare with the fears of parents who see their child critically ill. Grief may be displayed in many ways, and professional staff must respond sensitively, even when belligerence is encountered. Explanations may be resisted for a number of reasons, but the avenues of communication must be kept open.

Documentation

This aspect of care has been highlighted by many authors (e.g. Cetrulo and Cetrulo, 1989; James, 1991; McRae, 1993), especially with regard to potential litigation. The UKCC (1998) stresses the importance of maintaining good records, and Cohn (1984) notes that 'good record keeping is the single most useful thing that can be done to minimize risk, other than to talk with and take good care of patients'. This is particularly critical in the labour period, but refers to the woman's entire care from booking to postnatal check. In related research (Symon, 2000), a large proportion of midwives (and a smaller proportion of doctors) claimed to have improved their record-keeping as a result of the fear of litigation.

There is a standard litany about documentation in health care: entries in the case notes must be made at regular intervals, and these entries (including the countersigning signature) must be legible. While depressingly obvious, nevertheless in many cases in which there is a poor outcome even these minimum criteria have not been adhered to. The following is a checklist against such accusations:

- Detailed entries should be made in the notes, especially when a decision has been taken with regard to management. A lack of documentation in 'wait and see' decisions can make it appear as if no decision has been taken. This is best summed up by the adage: 'If you didn't write it, you didn't do it'. In one case a registrar was unable to recollect any of the events in question, and admitted that 'I would not necessarily make any comments in the notes if correct management was being followed'. In another case the failure on the part of the midwife to note any difficulty with a delivery led to the inference that excessive force had been used when Erb's palsy was diagnosed in the baby.
- Entries must be clear, accurate and legible. In one case there was considerable debate as to whether the obstetrician had written 'bladder' or 'bleeder' in an operation note. In another there were three different versions of the baby's Apgar scores, which did little to convey a sense of competence. What is written must also be logical. One midwife included what are apparently two mutually exclusive statements in her admission note: 'No SRM ... black substance in the vagina.' The expert report concluded that the midwife's actions were not those of a competent professional, the black substance

evidently being meconium. The nature (e.g. colour, whether fresh or old) and amount of meconium, when present, ought to be documented, together with information about the liquor. Although the presence of meconium does not necessarily indicate fetal compromise, this conclusion has been drawn (e.g. Wisniewski *v.* Central Manchester HA [1996]). Great care must be taken to document the relevant management decisions in these circumstances.

- Entries should be made contemporaneously. When this is not possible, they should be made as soon as is practicable. Memory recall will not be aided when there are gaps in the case notes, for whatever reason. In one case the midwife noted in her report: 'Fetal heart listened with sonicaid – satisfactory – I did not record it as the notes were in the other corner of the room and Mrs K needed me next to her all the time'. In such a situation, staff must make their entries promptly. Having notepaper to hand, and writing times and information (such as fetal heart rates) down as an *aide-mémoire* will help.
- Documentation must be stored effectively. A number of cases refer to partially or completely missing case notes, and there has been the inference that notes are sometimes lost deliberately as a stalling tactic by hospitals (Beech, 1990). In fact when case notes are missing, a defence is much harder to organize. Doherty (1986) notes that 'accurate note taking ... is the best preventative to, and defence from, legal action'. James (1991, p. 38) similarly notes that 'claims have become indefensible because this vital piece of evidence {the CTG} was missing ...'. Because a particular problem in litigation has been missing or deficient CTG traces, it is vital that midwives also record the fetal heart rate in the woman's case notes. Bear in mind that many legal actions are not raised for several years (in many cases involving cerebral palsy there is effectively no time limit), and because the paper on which CTG traces are printed is heat- and light-sensitive and is liable to tearing, it must be protected securely. Some units have introduced a sturdy envelope (for CTG traces only) that can be attached inside the case notes. Entries relating to rate and variability, as well as accelerations and decelerations, will help to clarify the record of this important marker of the fetal condition in the event that the CTG trace is unavailable.

Case records will be relied upon heavily in a legal investigation; given the unexpected nature of many legal claims, staff who fail to keep clear contemporaneous records, particularly in the labour ward, are courting danger. It may be difficult to maintain a good standard of record keeping when the unit is extremely busy or when emergencies occur, but there is a clear duty to make adequate entries in the case notes as soon as is practicable. This will assist any retrospective enquiry, in particular by helping the relevant staff members to recall particular sequences of events.

Cardiotocography

Cardiotocographs feature prominently in analyses of poor outcomes, and are a critical factor in many of the most emotive legal actions. In cases involving cerebral palsy the CTG may be crucial in determining whether the handicap is related to the intrapartum period, and, if so, whether staff reacted appropriately to signs of fetal compromise. It is vital for employers to ensure that all staff called upon to interpret CTG traces are competent to do so. Minimizing poor outcomes is the aim of good care, but there is a financial incentive too, since such cases are at the very top of the league of damages awards in clinical negligence. One of the cases under review here was settled for over £?m

Sadly, practitioners have in the past been placed in a position for which they are not prepared, as in this case where the defence noted:

> *[The midwife] admitted quite freely that she spent many hours in watching a fetal heart monitor which she was insufficiently trained to interpret or understand at the time. She has since been better trained and, looking back at the fetal heart traces during the period she was on duty, she sees them as being abnormal. In my opinion, quite a bit of liability must therefore attach to a system which asked midwives to watch a monitor which they are insufficiently trained to understand.*

In-service education is the standard means of ensuring this – Murphy *et al.* (1990) called for this to be mandatory, and Drife (1995) suggested 'regular training sessions on fetal monitoring' for midwives as part of a checklist for risk reduction. This is a minimum requirement: if attendance at a fire lecture can be mandatory in an attempt to reduce risk, then regular in-service training sessions on CTG use and interpretation must be mandatory for practitioners who use this technology. However, it was worrying to find in a large-scale survey of obstetricians and midwives (Symon, 1998b) that 65 per cent of the obstetricians felt that training for midwives was deficient in this regard, and indeed many midwives agreed with this. This must be a matter for concern, for it is the midwife who will usually first pick up on possible problems. The legal (and emotional) consequences of failing to do so may be devastating.

One study of 64 legal cases found a number of complaints made about CTGs, which included unsatisfactory or missing traces, abnormalities being ignored or not noticed, and traces simply not being done. Of 11 in the latter category, the authors note that in three of them 'midwives were asked by a doctor to carry out CTG but forgot' (Ennis and Vincent, 1990). The importance of good communication between doctors and midwives has already been referred to. Other studies have identified problems with not noticing signs of fetal distress, or not taking appropriate action quickly when such signs were noticed (Capstick and Edwards, 1990).

When to monitor, and for how long, is crucial. Many units will have protocols or policies that give suggestions/instructions on when monitoring should be carried out. In general terms, the higher the woman's risk rating, the more likely monitoring will be needed. Sadly, this does not always take place. In one case, the expert report noted:

> *There is a period of 90 minutes ... when there was no CTG recording. This is an unacceptable situation where the patient has had a previous section, at 42 weeks with meconium staining, and with CTG abnormalities which are persistent and who was on oxytocin.*

This catalogue of at-risk factors apparently did not alert midwives to the need for extra vigilance, and they were heavily criticized for this. It is vital to ensure that the pregnant woman knows why she is being monitored, and consents to this. This relates again to the matter of effective communication. The question of whether staff can or should insist on monitoring in certain circumstances produced some interesting differences of opinion in related research (Symon, 1998b).

Difficulties may be encountered with monitoring when the baby is very active or is in an unfavourable position, or if polyhydramnios or obesity is present. In such circumstances midwives must document the difficulties that prevent effective monitoring. Failing to do so, especially if the CTG trace is subsequently mislaid, can lead to an inference that no attempt was made to monitor at all.

One study that examined problems with the CTG found that: 'in five the abnormality was noted, but no action was taken; the staff believed the machine to be faulty and so ignored the trace' (Vincent *et al.*, 1991). While it may be tempting to assume that equipment within maternity units is efficient and well maintained, in view of the legal cases concerning apparently defective machinery this is not a safe assumption. Obsolete monitors must be replaced, and those that are used must be maintained to an acceptable standard. This of course has cost implications, but must be more financially appealing than the prospect of paying out hundreds of thousands of pounds because monitoring was either deficient or not carried out at all.

Because the CTG is only one marker of the fetal condition, it is recommended that equipment for fetal blood sampling also be provided (Murphy *et al.*, 1990; Drife, 1995).

Conclusion

This chapter has referred to an apparent general rise in societal expectations, and noted that maternity care seems to be particularly implicated. While such a rise in expectations will be due to many factors, among these may be publicity about the advances in technology that have reduced mortality rates, and the prevalence of the image of the smiling, healthy baby. How much practitioners may be held to have contributed to this rise in expectations is a matter of debate, but certainly the perceived reality is that we must deal with people who expect more of the health service.

This rise in expectations has been accompanied by an increased demand for openness and accountability from healthcare professionals. Developments in the law that covers allegations of clinical negligence may make defending such allegations much harder. Certainly the privileged position of healthcare practitioners in the eyes of the law is under challenge, and less confidence may now be placed in the traditional Bolam/Hunter *v.* Hanley defence.

Against this backdrop of increased expectations and reduced certainty in the law, this chapter has noted a wide variety in the clinical circumstances by which women and their families become litigants. The multiple reasons for suing obstetricians and midwives (and others involved in perinatal care) at first present a bewildering catalogue of potential legal flashpoints. However, the diverse heads of claims mask the common features that underlie the origins of these poor outcomes, and these were addressed earlier in this chapter under 'Clinical implications'.

Training and supervision are an ongoing responsibility for employers, and in a multidisciplinary field such as maternity care present a particular challenge. However, failing to meet this challenge will certainly increase the likelihood of a poor outcome. Communication problems, both between practitioners and between practitioners and the women under their care, have been seen to create significant difficulties. Healthcare professionals may be assumed to be intelligent individuals, but some evidently fail to maintain effectual communication channels, especially when things do not go well. Paradoxically, this is just when communication must be effective.

Just as some practitioners at times fail to communicate well, so a proportion of them continue to keep inadequate records. While the need to do so is well recognized, and many midwives claim to have improved their documentation as a result of the fear of litigation, deficiencies in this aspect of care remain, and provide a significant obstacle to rebutting an allegation of negligence. Competence in the interpretation of cardiotocographs also featured significantly in the analysis of legal claims. While the provision of training in this skill is mandatory in many units, it is also the responsibility of the practitioner to ensure that he or she is sufficiently trained and experienced before undertaking such duties. The law, after all, holds that practitioners are accountable for what they do.

While one of the aims of the civil law is to deter negligence, it is impossible to measure its deterrent effect. The theoretical deterrence of the tort/delict system has come in for some heavy criticism in recent years for a number of reasons, not least its questionable effectiveness in ensuring good practice. Practitioners who only practise safely because they fear legal involvement undermine the spirit of professionalism in health care. The promotion of health demands much more than such an approach. Practitioners work within a 'legal environment' – there are legal duties to provide a certain standard of care – and it is not denied that there is an incentive to try and avoid adversarial legal entanglement. However, risk management, while undoubtedly reactive in the sense that it has responded to the experience of litigation, is essentially a proactive clinical tool. While it aims to minimize exposure to litigation, its principal goal is the reduction of poor outcomes.

Neither risk management nor the civil law can guarantee the right to a perfect baby. In maternity care we are faced with high expectations, and a demand for openness and explanation when things do not go according to plan. While things go wrong for many different reasons, there are features common to many such outcomes. Practitioners have a responsibility to remain updated: we must be aware both of what others do, and of what constitutes good safe evidence-based practice. Promoting good care requires a constant review process, for our care and our standards are continually under scrutiny.

References

Acheson, D. (1991). Are obstetrics and midwifery doomed? *Midwives' Chronicle*, **104**, 158–66.

Anon (1990). Medical negligence: Hunter *v.* Hanley 35 years on. *Scots Law Times*, 325–7.

Anon (1997a). Bereaved family face legal fight. *The Herald*, **31 May**, 9.

Anon (1997b). Former midwives' leader pays £0.8m damages for baby with cerebral palsy. *Nursing Standard*, **11(22)**, 8.

Avis, M., Bond, M. and Arthur, A. (1997). Questioning patient satisfaction: an empirical investigation in two outpatient clinics. *Social Sci. Med.*, **44**, 85–92.

Bastian, H. (1990). Obstetrics and litigation: a consumer perspective. *Med. J. Aust.*, **153**, 340–45.

Beard, R. and O'Connor, A. (1995). Implementation of audit and risk management: a protocol. In: *Clinical Risk Management* (C. Vincent, ed.), pp. 350–74. BMJ Publishing Group.

Beaton, J. and Gupton, A. (1990). Childbirth expectations: a qualitative analysis. *Midwifery*, **6**, 133–9.

Beech, B. (1990). Accountability and compensation. *AIMS Q. J.*, **2(4)**, 1–3.

Black, N. (1990). Medical litigation and the quality of care. *Lancet*, **335**, 35–7.

Brazier, M. (1987). *Medicine, Patients, and the Law.* Penguin.

Capstick, J. B. and Edwards, P. (1990). Trends in obstetric malpractice claims. *Lancet*, **336**, 931–2.

Cetrulo, C. and Cetrulo, L. (1989). The legal liability of the medical consultant in pregnancy. *Med. Clin. North Am.*, **73(3)**, 557–65.

Clothier, C. (1989). Medical negligence and no-fault liability *Lancet*, **333**, 603–5.

Clow, K., Kurtz, D. and Ozment, J. (1996). Managing customer expectations of restaurants: an empirical study. *J. Restaurant Foodservice Marketing*, **1(3-04)**, 135–59.

Cohn, S. (1984). The nurse-midwife: malpractice and risk management. *J. Nurse-Midwifery*, **29**, 316–21.

Copperfield, T. (1996). Taking the law into your own hands. *Doctor*, **9 May**, 72–3.

Dann, G. (1996). Tourists' images of a destination – an alternative analysis. *J. Travel Tourism Marketing*, **5(1/2)**, 41–55.

Department of Health (1991). *Arbitration for Medical Negligence in the National Health Service.* HMSO.

Diamond, E. (1980). The deformed child's right to life. In: *Death, Dying and Euthanasia* (D. Horan and D. Mall, eds), University Publications of America.

Dillner, L. (1995). Babies' deaths linked to suboptimal care. *Br. Med. J.*, **310**, 757.

Dimond, B. (1996). Legal issues. The midwife as expert witness. *Modern Midwife*, **6(4)**, 22–3.

Dineen, M. (1996). Clinical risk management – a pragmatic approach. *Br. J. Midwifery*, **4**, 586–9.

Dingwall, R. (1994). Litigation and the threat to medicine. In: *Challenging Medicine* (J. Gabe and G. Williams, eds), pp. 46–64. Routledge.

Dingwall, R., Fenn, P. and Quam, L. (1991). *Medical Negligence – A Review and Bibliography.* Oxford Centre for Socio-Legal Studies.

Doherty, R. (1986). Childbirth: a natural process? *J. MDU*, **2(2)**, 10.

Doherty, R. and James, C. (1994). Malpractice in obstetrics and gynaecology. In: *Recent Advances in Obstetrics and Gynaecology* (J. Bonnar, ed.), No. 18, pp. 91–106. Churchill Livingstone.

Drife, J. O. (1995). Risk reduction in obstetrics. In: *Clinical Risk Management* (C. Vincent, ed.), pp. 129–46. BMJ Publishing Group.

Dyer, C. (1990). Pressure for no fault on three fronts. *Br. Med. J.*, **301**, 1010.

Dyer, C. (1995). Pilot study could cut medical negligence costs. *Br. Med. J.*, **311**, 770–71.

Easterbrook, J. (1996). Medical negligence update. *Solicitors' J.*, **140**, 381–2.

Ellis, J. (1988). Doctors in training: who bears the cost? In: *Medical Negligence: Addressing the Issues*, Medical Protection Society.

Ennis, M. and Vincent, C. (1990). Obstetric accidents: a review of 64 cases. *Br. Med. J.*, **300**, 1365–7.

Fenn, P. and Dingwall, R. (1995). Mutual trust? *Br. Med. J.*, **310**, 756.

Foster, C. (1996). Causation in medical negligence cases: recent developments. *Solicitors' J.*, **140**, 1098–100.

Fresco, A. (2000). Father used half of son's £40000 payout. *The Times*, **9 Mar**.

Genn, H. (1999). *Mediation in Action.* Calouste Gulbenkian Foundation.

Goldrein, I. (1994). Exploding the Bolam myth. *New Law J.*, **Sep 16–Oct 28**, pp. 1237–1481.

Ham, C., Dingwall, R. and Fenn, P. (1988). *Medical Negligence: Compensation and Accountability.* King's Fund Institute.

Henderson, M. (1997). Baby died after doctor used forceps ten times. *The Times*, **21 Nov**, p. 8.

Hodgson, J. (1981). Professional negligence clarified. *New Law J.*, **131**, 2.

Howie, R. (1983). The standard of care in medical negligence. *Juridical Rev.*, **28**, 193–223.

James, C. (1991). Risk management in obstetrics and gynaecology. *J. MDU*, **7**, 36–8.

Kerson, T. (1994). Field instruction in social work settings: a framework for teaching. *Clin. Supervisor*, **12**, 1–31.

Klein, R. (1973). *Complaints against Doctors.* C. Knight.

Lamont, L. (1993). Why patients don't sue doctors. *J. MDU*, **9**, 39–41.

Lindsay, Y. (1994). Personal view: 'Why don't you sue?'. *Br. Med. J.*, **308**, 1377.

Maternal and Child Health Research Consortium (1997*). Confidential Enquiry into Stillbirths and Deaths in Infancy*, 4th Report. MCHRC.

McKain, D. (2000). Woman loses action over birth *Herald*, **27 Apr.**

McRae, M. (1993). Litigation, electronic fetal monitoring, and the obstetric nurse. *J. Obstet. Gynecol. Neonatal Nursing*, **22**, 416–419.

Medical Protection Society (1989). *Annual Report.* Medical Protection Society.

Murphy, K., Johnson, P., Moorcraft, J. *et al.* (1990). Birth asphyxia and the intrapartum cardiotoco-graph. *Br. J. Obstet. Gynaecol.*, **97**, 470–79.

Norrie, K. (1985). Medical negligence: who sets the standard? *J. Med. Ethics*, **11**, 135–7.

O'Meara, C. (1993). An evaluation of consumer perspectives of childbirth and parenting education. *Midwifery*, **9**, 210–19.

Saunders, P. (1992). Recruitment in obstetrics and gynaecology: RCOG sets initiatives. *Br. J. Obstet. Gynaecol.*, **99**, 538–46.

Scott, W. (1998). Bolam and Bolitho: a new standard of care for doctors? *New Law J.*, **148**, 64.

Shank, M. and Hayes, T. (1995). Understanding professional service expectations: do we know what our students expect in a quality education? *J. Prof. Services Marketing*, **13**, 71–89.

Symon, A. (1998a). Perinatal litigation – expectations: can we meet them? *Br. J. Midwifery*, **6**, 330–33.

Symon, A. (1998b). *Litigation – The Views of Midwives and Obstetricians.* Hochland and Hochland.

Symon, A. (1999). Perinatal litigation in Scotland, 1980–95: its incidence, rate and nature. *J. Obstet. Gynaecol.*, **19**, 239–47.

Symon, A. (2000). Litigation and defensive clinical practice: quantifying the problem. *Midwifery*, **16**, 8–14.

Symon, A. (2001). *Obstetric Litigation from A–Z.* Quay Books.

Tharmaratnam, S. and Gillmer, M. (1995). The litigation boom in obstetrics. *Obst. Gynaecol. Today*, **6(2)**, 17–20.

United Kingdom Central Council for Nursing, Midwifery and Health Visiting (1998). *Guidelines for Records and Record Keeping.* UKCC.

Vincent, C., Martin, T. and Ennis, M. (1991). Obstetric accidents: the patient's perspective. *Br. J. Obstet. Gynaecol.*, **98**, 390–95.

Vincent, C., Young, M. and Phillips, A. (1994). Why do people sue doctors? A study of patients and relatives taking legal action. *Lancet*, **343**, 1609–13.

Warden, J. (1996). NHS repeats its mistakes. *Br. Med. J.*, **312**, 1247.

Woolf, Lord (Chairman) (1996). *Access to Justice.* Final Report to the Lord Chancellor on the Civil Justice System in England and Wales. Lord Chancellor's Department.

Legal cases:

Barnett *v.* Chelsea HMC [1968]1 All England Reports 1068.

Bolam *v.* Friern HMC [1957] 2 All England Reports 118.

Bolitho *v.* City & Hackney HA [1993] 4 Medical Law Reports, 381.

Corley *v.* North West Hertfordshire Health Authority [1997] 8 Medical Law Reports, 45–56.

Donoghue *v.* Stevenson [1932] Session Cases (House of Lords) 31, 1932 Scots Law Times 317.

Dowdie *v.* Camberwell Health Authority [1997] 8 Medical Law Reports, 368–376.

Gaughan *v.* Bedfordshire Health Authority [1997] 8 Medical Law Reports, 182–190.

Hunter *v.* Hanley [1955] Session Cases 200.

Maynard *v.* West Midlands RHA [1984] 1 WLR 634.

Robertson *v.* Nottingham Health Authority [1997] 8 Medical Law Reports, 1–15.

Rolland *v.* Lothian Health Board, 1981 (unreported).

Sidaway *v.* Board of Governors of the Bethlem Royal Hospital and others [1984] 2 WLR 778, CA; [1985] 1 All E.R. 643.

Whitehouse *v.* Jordan and another [1981] 1 WLR 246 (H.L.); [1980] 1 All England Reports 650 C.A.

Wisniewski *v.* Central Manchester Health Authority [1996] 7 Medical Law Reports, 248–265.

4

Intra- and inter-professional behaviour and communication

Monica Thompson

Communication is like a piece of driftwood on a sea of conflicting currents. Sometimes the shore will be littered with debris, sometimes again it will be bare. The amount and direction of movement is not aimless and indirectional, but is a response to all the forces — winds, tides and currents – which come into play.

(Jay M. Jackson)

Introduction

Communication is an essential and natural component of daily living that we engage in unconsciously. Communication failures, however, can have a direct or indirect impact on outcome. In maternity care, whilst the full impact of communication failure on perinatal loss may be difficulty to assess, it remains a recurring issue in recent reports on the Maternity Services in the United Kingdom (Audit Commission, 1997; DOH, 1998; MCHRC, 2000). There are regular problems with the standard of communication in general; with giving conflicting advice to women; the standard, amount and types of information given; the problems caused when information is misunderstood; and the need to debrief women. Finally, there is a need to determine the extent to which inter-professional working and communication between professionals and with women impact on outcomes. The most recent *Confidential Enquiry into Stillbirths and Deaths in Infancy* (MCHRC, 2000) cites communication failure in 17 per cent of comments analysed in the enquiries into intrapartum-related deaths. This prompted the Maternal and Child Health Research Consortium to commission a review of published evidence of the contribution of these failures to perinatal loss. The *Confidential Enquiry into Stillbirths and Deaths in Infancy*, however, reflects an acceptance that medical science and technology has the ability to improve perinatal outcomes. It persists in examining perinatal and post-neonatal deaths by systematic scientific enquiry. The biomedical model that underpins the MCHRC's prevention agenda has been roundly challenged recently. Fowler (2000) feels the narrow medical paradigm within which it operates only serves to maintain a threatened medical profession's stronghold on childbirth. It is not a stronghold women want or midwives should embrace; nor is it in keeping with the government's agenda for primary care-led maternity services. MCHRC sustains a downstream approach, focusing on changing individual lifestyles and behaviours in the belief that advice and information derived from superior medical knowledge must be followed (Ewles and Simmett, 1990). In its many recommendations for practice concerning communication, it highlights the evidence that communication failures often occur at times of handover of care and recommends that systems should be put in place to ensure that information transfer is complete and accurate (MCHRC, 2000). Clearly then, where communication, from whatever source, is poor and the outcome sub-optimal, the fundamental expectation of parents, let alone the 'right to a perfect baby', has been compromised. Communication plays a pivotal role here.

This chapter explores the nature, quality and quantity of inter- and intra-professional interactions, behaviours and communication within the various contexts of maternity care, and the intrapartum care setting in particular. It outlines the general principles of effective communication, and then examines the power of language and its social constructs in the labour suite. It goes on to discuss the concept of authoritative knowledge and the transfer of information and the relationship this has on subsequent decision-making. Finally, the implications of these issues are discussed with respect to the formulation and implementation of woman-centred maternity care within new service delivery models, and of multi-professional teaching and learning opportunities within educational institutions. Questions are raised throughout the chapter, such as how is knowledge legitimated (and by whom)? How are risk and safety in childbirth perceived and evaluated? Who are the gatekeepers of information? How is information communicated and disseminated? How are professional autonomy and inter-professionalism reconciled?

Effective communication

Effective communication requires clarity of thought, focus of mind and the necessity of being thoroughly conversant with the subject matter. It remains something of a paradox, however, that whenever words and their diverse meanings are concerned, doubt and confusion are also often highly conspicuous (Brown, 1958; Spender, 1980; Tannen, 1992).

> *I know you think you understand what you thought I said, but I'm not sure what you heard is what I meant.*
>
> (Hewison, 1997)

This statement, often used in communication training sessions, illustrates awareness that communication is a complex process fraught with difficulty.

Janner (1988) contends that communication demands the three essential Es – energy, enthusiasm and excitement; boredom is its enemy. Communication is not only the sharing of thoughts, it is also the ever-changing process of sending and receiving messages that result in the creation of a reciprocal relationship. Whether writing, speaking, trying to persuade, inform, entertain, explain, convince or elucidate, we always have four general objectives:

– *To be received (heard or read);*
– *to be understood;*
– *to be accepted; and*

– to get action (change of behaviour or attitude).

When we fail to achieve any of these, we have failed to communicate.
(Stanton, 1990, p.1)

Alder and Rodman (1994) believe that the key to successful communication is to share an adequate amount of information in a skilful manner. They contend that, rather like athletic ability, even the most inept of us can learn to be more effective with training and practice, and those who are talented can always become better. Organizations are dependent upon effective communication routes. They are the veins and arteries carrying the organization's lifeblood (Evans, 1990).

'Organizational' communication refers to the communication used to promote social organization through the co-ordination of interdependent groups. This encompasses interpersonal, intra-professional and group communication. Kings (1990) maintains that shared information is critical in accomplishing organizational goals as it provides members with rationale and direction for co-ordinating their activities. In modern healthcare systems this is translated through the healthcare team, an integrated multidisciplinary unit working collaboratively to provide quality healthcare services. Health care today is no simple matter involving single clinicians and individual patients/clients; care is more often provided by multiprofessionals in complex institutions, utilizing several layers of support, consultation and referral. This is particularly evident in the labour suites of many hospitals, promoting a variety of intrapartum care options.

Communication in health care

The healthcare team functions along a continuum from parallel practice to the cohesive inter-professional team (Figure 4.1)

It is only as groups of professionals meet regularly in each other's presence, around specific goals, that the inter-professional team emerges. Common goals, co-operative relationships and co-ordinated activities are ideally the hallmarks of all collaborative professionals' work. It is when professionals meet together to pursue these activities that a health and social care support system, which is greater than the sum of its professionals, is created – i.e. the inter-professional healthcare support system.

The effectiveness of healthcare teams, however, depends on the quality of communication among team members (Wise, 1974; Thornton, 1978). It is well

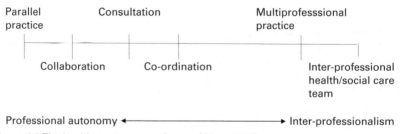

Figure 4.1 The healthcare team continuum (Glen, 1997).

documented that the more competent communication is between members of healthcare teams, the more likely they are to provide 'therapeutic' communication, social support, satisfaction, information exchange and co-operation. Alternatively, the less competent communication is, the more likely they are to provide 'pathological' communication, lack of social support, dissatisfaction, information barriers and lack of co-operation (Evans, 1990).

Intentions are communicated not only by the language used but also through an extensive repertoire of body gestures. In the context of midwifery, good communication plays a vital role in determining choice and positively assists in decision-making between professional carers and women. Poor communication, on the other hand, heightens uncertainty, selectively informs and so effectively conceals available options (Stapleton, 1997). Making care options available encourages participation and shifts the decision-making process from professionals to women. Women are encouraged to articulate their needs in the hope that there are clear options available to them. However, as evidenced in the Changing Childbirth pilots, when a cost-neutral government policy prevails, real choice and by extension real change are severely compromised (Rosser, 1997).

Numerous government reports and recent research (Audit Commission, 1993, 1998; DoH, 1993, Scottish Office Home and Health Department, 1993) all emphasize the need for improved communication between care providers and childbearing women. Women's priorities in their care suggest that good information and communication are among the most important aspects of maternity care. In a study by Drew *et al.* (1989), women were asked to score 40 aspects of maternity care on a scale from essential to irrelevant. Women put 'the baby being healthy' at the top of the list, followed by two communication issues; 'doctors talking to you in a way you understand' and 'having all your questions answered by staff'. However, other studies that have used observation of labour care have shown that women's attempts to find out what is happening are sometimes ignored or diverted by responses from midwives that sterilize the communication (Kirkham, 1989; Garcia and Garford, 1990). More recently, Hunt and Symonds (1995) in their ethnographic study on the social meaning of midwifery concluded:

> *The study has demonstrated that the key issues of control, continuity and choice were in essence issues in communication. The women at Valley Maternity Hospital were without doubt rendered powerless by the system. The communication patterns were established in order to further the main goal of 'getting through the work'. Whilst the midwives were supportive, kind and technically proficient, the site of the birth process has reduced this critical life event to a production line system. Communication was the major issue that coloured the quality of the birth experience for most women.*

Central tenets of all communication are language, knowledge and power, and these cannot be disentangled. This is so much so that Hugman (1991) claims that the power of the professional is based on the control of language and the knowledge that rests with that professional. Language and the terminology used, which conveys social meaning, are the determinants of the relationship between midwives and women on the one hand, and midwives and medical men on the other. These will now be explored.

The power of language

The language we use is an expression of our values, attitudes and beliefs, which are culturally and socially determined (Duranti and Goodwin, 1992). Language assumes power by the identity, solidarity and status it conveys on groups within society (Todd and Fisher, 1988). Consequently, it is believed to be the most subtle and powerful technique we have of controlling others. Bastian (1992), Leap (1992) and Walton (1995) all make reference to the profusion of commonly used words and phrases that disempower and trivialize women. They claim that the language we use indicates not only where the balance of power lies, but also our own personal attitudes and the wider ideologies informing midwifery care. Examining the discourses and the power relations between childbearing women, midwives and obstetricians further demonstrates the controlling nature of language where 'privileged knowledge' is dominant (Oakley, 1984; Hewison, 1993). Hewison emphasizes the effect of medical language in care where medical terminologies associated with the concept of risk, for example 'incompetent cervix', 'intra-uterine growth retardation', 'failure to progress' and 'post-term', all serve to:

> ... reinforce a definition of pregnancy and birth as inherently hazardous and requiring medical intervention ... the term 'risk' evokes feelings and concerns to such an extent that it is accepted in a critical way that helps determine the delivery of maternity care. The term represents the way an idea or concept can be dominant purely through its suggested meaning.

Through this use of language, power is exerted to ensure that medical knowledge is legitimate. This then becomes the 'authoritative' knowledge.

Authoritative knowledge

The power of authoritative knowledge is not that it is correct, but that it counts. It is the knowledge that participants agree counts in a particular situation, that they see as consequential and the basis on which they make decisions and provide justifications for courses of action. Jordan (1997) observed that in American hospital births, medical knowledge supersedes and delegitimizes other potentially relevant sources of knowledge, such as the woman's prior experience and the knowledge she has of the state of her body. In contrast, however, she found that in the rural communities of the Yucaton, the store of knowledge required in conducting a birth is drawn from the shared history and the experience of all those in attendance – the woman's family, the midwife and the other experienced women in the community. Horizontal distribution of authoritative knowledge is evident here in the decision-making process.

Jordan's (1992) anthropological analysis of birth argues that obstetric technology and technical procedures are central to the labour ward environment, and that the 'ownership' of the artefacts necessary to manage the labour simultaneously defines and displays who should be seen as possessing authoritative knowledge and consequently as holding legitimate decision-making power. Throughout labour, the obstetric nurse looks at the external fetal monitor for information during the course of contractions (videotape evidence shows the obstetric nurse glancing at the machine often just when the woman is in greatest distress). In this setting, checking on the machine is not an occasional event but an ever-present phenomenon.

In this labour room, authoritative knowledge is privileged, the prerogative of the physician, without whose official certification of the woman's state the birth cannot proceed. The woman's knowledge of her body's readiness to 'push' counts for nothing. Only the doctor can confirm this and so legitimize this information. This fiction is maintained by all other attendants.

The gatekeeping function of the physician is fulfilled when he or she pronounces when pushing can commence and so effectively determines when the second stage begins. Furthermore, reserving certification to the physician assures that the birth does not proceed without him or her. This artificial punctuation of the labour process skews the length of second stage in the direction of shortening the normal stages of labour. Whilst this is not intended to indict all American hospital births, it does serve to illustrate what happens when technology–birth dependent knowledge becomes hierarchically distributed (Jordan, 1992). Similar medical models of care prevail in UK maternity care settings, where doctors' professional dominance sees childbirth as a mechanistic, scientific problem to be solved (Hunt and Symonds, 1995).

Labour ward behaviours

Doctors' unquestioned status and authority rests in the social contract that accords them that authority. This authority is not only visible in the ritual deference paid to the superior status of medical knowledge, but also in the behaviour of other professionals and the way activities in the labour ward are orchestrated. The kind of 'framing' by other team members, as observed, is not restricted to the labour room, but is common in various medical interactions that have staff of various rank present. Kirkham (1989), observing labours in hierarchical hospital settings in the UK notes staff 'waiting on' the doctors in what she calls a pattern of 'dancing attendance'.

How then does this behaviour and the interaction between midwives and obstetricians influence decision-making and the quality of care delivered? In the past the relations between midwives and doctors have been highly charged and traditionally antagonistic (Donnison, 1977). It is acknowledged that professional relationships between midwifery and medical colleagues are influenced by social, political, historical and educational factors, and so can be very difficult (Drife, 1993 and Green *et al.*, 1994). However, the recent national survey of women's views of maternity care would suggest that improvements in communication and relationships have taken place (Audit Commission, 1997). Nevertheless, barriers still exist between obstetricians and midwives and between midwives and women. Little attention had been paid to this interface, with the exception of Walker (1976) and Kirkham (1989), prior to the study undertaken by Wallace *et al.* (1995). This prospective observational study examined the quality and quantity of midwife–doctor referrals in the intrapartum setting in a large tertiary referral maternity hospital. Of the 204 midwife-led cases examined during the study period, 90 (44 per cent) required medical intervention for reasons concerning failure to progress, fetal distress and need for analgesia. Whilst generally the nature of the referral was deemed appropriate by 67 per cent of medical staff, the cited examples and comments regarding inappropriate referrals would suggest a fundamental misconception of the midwives' role, and their responsibility regarding referral on detection of a deviation from the norm. (Rule 40, *Midwives' Rules and Code of Practice, 1998*). Comments by obstetric senior house officers (SHOs) included 'midwives try to tell you your job'; 'midwives distrust new SHOs'; and 'midwives tend to bottle out from taking responsibility'. Senior midwives referred directly to registrars in regard to midwife-led cases. The mismatch between the hierarchy of skill of midwives and hierarchy of status of SHOs as discussed by Kitzinger *et al.* (1990) was evident here, where subtle manipulation of SHOs occurred. It is believed that these referral practices not only undermine the learning opportunities for junior house officers, but also curtail the important role experienced midwives play in this activity.

Relationships with other professionals

It further challenges the preservation of professional autonomy and dominance if expertise and knowledge is shared in a collaborative, supportive way. The minimization of professional autonomy produces a certain continuous level of tension in the inter-professional health and social care team. As Glen (1997; unpublished) contends, if members diminish the uniqueness of their professional base of knowledge, values and skills, their contributions to the goals of the team – effective, holistic health care – are diminished. If, on the other hand, members maintain professional differences too strongly, the internal functioning of the team can be impaired. Other investigators, however, have noted mechanisms that professionals can use to emphasize similarities without diluting uniqueness. These mechanisms include:

* Common orientation to the client/patient as the primary unit of attention
* Similarities in treatment modalities
* Common bodies of knowledge
* Shared language
* Shared status and position.

Competencies for health professionals of the future will include (Larson, 1995):

* Collaborative competence
* Public health focus
* Expanded accountability
* Appropriate use of technology
* Cost-effective care
* Prevention/promotion of healthy lifestyles
* Patient and family involvement in decision-making
* Information management
* Orientation to life-long learning.

The latest strategy document from the Royal College of Midwives, *Vision 2000*, reflects many of these mechanisms. However, it also recognizes that hierarchical cultures, professional territorialism, established organizational habits, and understaffing all pose a real challenge to midwives and managers seeking to establish women-centred services where there is reluctance to change from service-centred provision. This document, like many before it, calls for one-to-one midwifery care in labour, a situation not experienced in many maternity units throughout the country. Yet it is claimed to be the only intervention proven to improve birth outcome, increase maternal satisfaction and reduce the need for expensive intervention (Audit Commission, 1997; RCOG and RCM 1998; RCM, 2000).

Conclusion

Communication failure is the most commonly voiced criticism of health care in general. Effective communication is a complex reciprocal process. It requires clarity of thought, and the possession of relevant information so that we are received, understood, accepted, and achieve action. Arguably it is the lifeblood of an organization. This is particularly so in modern maternity services, which are dependent upon integrated, multidisciplinary work units.

In analysing communication and inter-professional relations, it is clear that the use of language, knowledge and positional power are tightly woven components. In the past, privileged stances have been adopted by the dominant professional and have fuelled the power struggle between midwives and medical men. Now, however, the ideology of women empowerment is accepted and valued, forcing professionals to re-examine their power positions and re-focus their respective contributions to women's reproduction health.

Nevertheless, the values implicit in professionalization have led midwives to take on the values of the dominant obstetricians emphasizing technical skill. Expertise and professionalism are often confused. The former is something to be worked for and shared, while the latter is elitist, exclusive, sexist, racist and classist (Ehrenreich and English, 1973).

Midwifery has had traditional relationships with medicine that have been enabling for doctors. Deference and working by proxy, as described by Kitzinger *et al.* (1990) and more recently by Wallace *et al.* (1995), are still observed among the strategies employed by midwives to achieve a desired outcome. The challenge now is to develop relationships that are enabling for midwives and women. We need to develop the 'emotional labour' of care, ensuring that the research that shows how social support as distinct from clinical care improves outcome is widely implemented.

The evidence from the plethora of government reports and commissioned research outlined earlier in the chapter perhaps offers few new solutions to the questions posed. The old paradigm where information is selectively communicated, medical dominance and autonomy prevail, and midwives practise deference and work by proxy, has effectively shifted. Fundamentally, the variable distribution in perinatal mortality and morbidity and so the challenge to the expectation for a 'perfect baby' is directly related to the inequalities in health between the most and least privileged sections of society. It is now recognized that a public health model of primary care has much to contribute to the determination of risk and safety in childbirth. It also requires a restructuring of our definition of childbirth as a natural and social event, with its risks being mainly social and economic in origin (Fowler, 2000).

Shared learning opportunities for healthcare professionals is still sporadic and not universal. The call for stronger commitment by our educational institutions to take seriously the task of educating for professional pluralism is welcomed.

This will help minimize differences, arrogance and dominance without diluting professional uniqueness.

These initiatives, together with implementing the practice recommendations from MCHRC (2000) and RCOG and RCM (1998), will go a considerable way towards reconciling inter- and intra-professional tensions and so maximizing optimal perinatal outcome. The right then to a 'perfect baby' may be realized.

References

Alder, R.B. and Rodman, G. (1994). *Understanding Human Communication*, 5th edn. Harcourt Brace College Distributors.

Audit Commission (1993). *What seems to be the Matter: Communication Between Hospital Patients*. HMSO.

Audit Commission (1997). *First Class Delivery: Improving Maternity Services in England and Wales*. Audit Commisison publications.

Audit Commission (1998). *First Class Delivery: A National Survey of Women's Views of Maternity Care*. Belmont Press.

Bastian, H. (1992). Confined, managed and delivered: the language of obstetrics. *Br. J. Obstet. Gynaecol.*, **99**, 92–3.

Brown, R. (1958). *Words and Things; An Introduction to Language*. Free Press.

Department of Health (1993). *Changing Childbirth. Report of the Expert Maternity Group*. HMSO.

Department of Health (1998). *Why Mothers Die – Report on Confidential Enquiries into Maternal Deaths in the United Kingdom 1994–1996*. HMSO.

Donnison, J. (1977). *Midwives and Medical Men: A History of Interprofessional Rivalries and Women's Rights*. Heinemann.

Drew, N. C., Salmon, P. and Webb, L. (1989). Mothers', midwives' and obstetricians' views on the features of obstetric care which influence satisfaction with childbirth. *Br. J. Obstet. Gynaecol.*, **96**, 1084–8.

Drife, J. O. (1993). Errors and accidents in obstetrics. In: *Medical Accidents* (C. Vincent, M. Ennis and R. J. Audley, eds), pp. 34–51. Oxford University Press.

Duranti, A. and Goodwin, C. (1992). *Rethinking Context: Language as an Intervention Phenomenon*. Cambridge University Press.

Ehrenreich, B. and English, D. (1973). *Witches, Midwives and Nurses: A History of Women Healers*, Glass Mountain Pamphlet. The Feminist Press.

Evans, D. W. (1990). *People, Communication and Organisations*, 2nd edn. Pitman Publications.

Ewles, L. and Simmett, J. (1990). *Promoting Health: A Practical Guide to Health Education*. J. Wiley & Sons.

Fowler, W. (2000). Focusing upstream to analyse perinatal workability roles. *Br. J. Midwifery*, **8(7)**, 415–20.

Garcia, J. and Garford, S. (1990). Parents and newborn babies in the labour ward. In: *The Politics of Maternity Care* (J. Garcia, M. Richards and R. Kilpatrick, eds). Oxford University Press.

Glen, S. (1997). *Shaping the Future of Nursing, Midwifery and Health Visiting Education in Scotland*. Unpublished conference paper.

Green, J., Kitzinger, J. and Coupland, V. (1994). Midwives' responsibilities, medical staffing, structures and women's choices in childbirth. In: *Midwives, Research and Childbirth*, Vol. 3 (S. Robinson and A. M. Thomson, eds), pp. 5–29. Chapman and Hall.

Hewison, A. (1993). The language of labour: an examination of the discourses on childbirth. *Midwifery*, **9**, 225–34.

Hewison, A. (1997). The language of management and enduring challenge. *J. Nursing Management*, **5**, 133–41.

Hugman, R. (1991). *Power in Caring Professions*. Macmillan.

Hunt, S. and Symonds, A. (1995). *The Social Meaning of Midwifery*. Macmillan.

Janner, G. (1988). *Janner on Communication*. Hutchison Business Books.

Jordan, B. (1992). Technology and social interaction: notes on the achievement of authoritative knowledge in complex settings. In: *IRL Technical Report IRL 92-0027*. Palo Alto, California: Institute of Research on Learning.

Jordan, B. (1997) Authoritative knowledge and its constructions. In: *Childbirth and Authoritative Knowledge – Cross-Cultural Perspectives* (R. Davis-Floyd and C. F. Sargent, eds). University of California Press.

Kings, G. L. (1990). *Organisational Communication: Theory and Practice*, 2nd edn. Longman.

Kirkham, M. J. (1989). Midwives and information-giving during labour. In: *Midwives, Research and Childbirth*, Vol. 1 (S. Robinson and A. M. Thomson, eds). Chapman and Hall.

Kitzinger, J., Green, J. and Coupland, V. (1990). Labour relations: midwives and doctors on the labour ward. In: *The Politics of Maternity Care* (J. Garcia, R. Kilpatrick and M. Richards, eds). Clarendon Press.

Larson, E. (1995). New rules for the game – interdisciplinary education for health professionals. *Nursing Outlook*, **43(4)**, 180–81.

Leap, N. (1992). The power of words. *Nursing Times*, **88(21)**, 60–61.

Maternal and Child Health Research Consortium (2000). *Confidential Enquiry into Stillbirths and Deaths in Infancy*, 7th Report. MCHRC.

Oakley, A. (1984). *The Captive Womb: A History of the Medical Care of Pregnant Women*. Basil Blackwell.

Rosser, J. (1997). Lies, damned lies and economics – counting the cost of maternity pilot schemes. *MIDIRS Midwifery Digest*, **7(2)**, 41–4.

Royal College of Midwives (2000) *Vision 2000*. RCM.

Royal College of Obstetricians and Gynaecologists, and Royal College of Midwives (1998) *Towards Safer Childbirth*. RCOG.

Scottish Office Home and Health Department (1993). *Health Policy and Public Health Directorate. Provision of Maternity Services in Scotland: A Policy Review*. HMSO.

Spender, D. (1980) *Man-made Language*. Routledge and Kegan Paul.

Stanton, N. (1990). *Communications*. Macmillan Press.

Stapleton, H. (1997). Choice in the face of uncertainty. In: *Reflections on Midwifery* (M. J. Kirkham and E. R. Perkins, eds). Baillière Tindall.

Tannen, D. (1992) *You Just Don't Understand: Woman and Men in Conversation*. Virago.

Thornton, K. C. (1978). *Health Care Teams as Multi Methodological Research: Communication Yearbook*. Transaction Press.

Todd, A. and Fisher, S. (1988). *Gender and Discourse: The Power of Talk*, Vol. 3. Ablex Publishing Corporation.

Walker, J. F. (1976). Midwife or obstetric nurse? Some perceptions of midwives and obstetricians on the role of the midwife. *J. Adv. Nursing.* **1,** 129–38.

Wallace, E. M., Mcintosh, C. L., Brownlee, M. *et al.* (1995). An observational study of midwife–medical staff interaction in a labour ward environment. *J. Obstet. Gynaecol.*, **15**, 165–70.

Walton, I. (1995). Words as symbols. *Modern Midwife*, **5(2)**, 35–6.

Wise, H. *et al.* (1974). *Making Health Teams Work*. Ballinger.

5

The roles of the midwifery manager and supervisor of midwives

Sue Stewart

Introduction

Risk management in the health service can be subdivided into three main areas; clinical, financial, and health and safety. In the past financial risk management was seen to be the most important element, but since the rise in litigation clinical risk management has now become as important.

This book concentrates on clinical risk management, but the other large element of risk management (health and safety) must not be forgotten as the two areas can impact on each other. Although health and safety risks are important, it is the clinical risks that will more frequently affect the midwife and so involve managers and supervisors of midwives as well.

This chapter explores the roles and responsibilities of, and the relationships between, the manager and supervisor of midwives in the clinical aspects of risk management. It identifies the perspectives of both roles and looks at their main emphases. Clinical risk management forms the basis of audit, and each member of the midwifery team has a distinct and collective part to play. This chapter seeks to clarify the roles of each member of the midwifery team and the relationships between the midwifery team and the woman and her partner during the process of childbirth. As midwifery practice has developed so too have midwifery management and supervision of midwives. How these developments have contributed to clinical management is also considered.

If clinical risk management is to be effective, the quality of care provided has to be continually reviewed and procedures that do not support good practice need to be addressed. Management of change is a difficult aspect of the manager's and the supervisor's roles, and needs to be handled sensitively. Good communication, with mutual respect and support between the manager and supervisor, can only benefit the clinical risk management process by ensuring competent, confident midwives who are committed to high quality care.

Risk management

Collins New English Dictionary (1997) defines risk as the possibility of incurring misfortune or loss. Therefore, although financial and clinical risk management are the major risk management concerns for the health service, the health and safety element of risk management must not be forgotten.

Health and safety risk management can be subdivided into the two main aspects of hospital activity: clinical and non-clinical.

Although this book looks at the impact of clinical risk management on maternity care, the roles of the midwifery manager and supervisor of midwives in connection with the health and safety aspects must not be overlooked. If the health and safety aspects of the environment are not addressed there can be an adverse affect on the care provided, thus affecting the clinical risk management. For example, a midwife who is unwell or overtired can contribute to poor quality care and so put the woman and Trust at risk. There is a responsibility for both manager and supervisor in both aspects of risk management, as one should not take precedence over the other. The fear of litigation has impacted on clinical risk management by insisting on procedures/protocols in the clinical as well as financial areas.

The term 'risk management' started to become high profile in the early 1990s. In 1993 the National Health Service Executive produced a manual for all Chief Executives of NHS Trust hospitals, giving guidance on risk management (DoH, 1993a), which prompted more NHS Trusts to take a proactive approach. At about the same time the United Kingdom Central Council (UKCC) revised the *Midwives' Rules* (UKCC, 1993) and the *Midwives' Code of Practice* (UKCC, 1994), making it mandatory for a supervisor of midwives to have completed an approved course of instruction prior to taking up the appointment.

The aim of risk management should be to improve the quality of the service and reduce the costs associated with litigation, these two elements being closely linked.

The purpose of supervision of midwifery is to 'safeguard and enhance the quality of care for the childbearing mother and her family' (ENB, 1996). Therefore, supervision should be seen as an integral part of clinical risk management.

The people involved

All managers, including clinical midwifery managers, supervisors of midwives, and midwives, have an essential role in the process. Good maternity care can only be delivered by effective teamwork. *Changing Childbirth* (DoH, 1993b) highlighted the parochial and territorial approach of professions and showed that they have been detrimental to maternity care. However, what about the client and her partner? If a Trust takes clinical risk management seriously, then the client and her partner must be considered as another important cog in the wheel. It is understandable why complaints can be viewed negatively, as they are costly in human resource time as well as in loss of professional confidence. However, it is because of this costly and inevitable process that they should be viewed positively and lessons learned. Clinical audit is valuable, but it does usually only take the professional stance, as most clinical audits are undertaken by clinicians to look at effectiveness of care. They may not take into account the patient's view of whether the treatment was beneficial, or whether it matched her expectations. Most complaints identify issues where the client's perspective is different from that of the clinician. If the concepts of choice, control and continuity in *Changing Childbirth* (DoH, 1993b) are to be developed and women's views are to be taken into account when developing services, then complaints cannot be ignored.

Many Trusts are now actively seeking the views of clients by customer satisfaction surveys and focus groups, and are positively seeking a cross-section of the local population to be representatives on the Maternity Services Liaison Committees. By seeking women's views, a maternity service can be developed and continually reviewed to ensure that it is in line with the needs of clients. Another way that clinical risk can be reduced is by taking a proactive approach. However, it must be remembered that in order for lay people to contribute to any debate with health professionals, support and possibly training will be required. For many members of the public a discussion with healthcare professionals can be very daunting, and so valuable contributions may be lost. If maternity service provision is to be truly equitable for all, it is essential to obtain views from representative members of the public. This includes those with social problems or physical disabilities, and those who do not have English as their first language. Some women in these groups may be less able to articulate their views in a multi-professional forum when compared with the stereotypical confident middle-class working woman, but their views are just as important.

The manager and clinical risk management

Clinical risk management should be an integral part of good management practice. It forms a basis of audit, which is essential if high quality care is to be provided. Technology, research and women's needs have developed and changed through the 1980s and 1990s, and have impacted on clinical care. For a high quality service to be provided, the care must take account of these changes and developments and therefore audit is essential. Problems or potential problems need to be identified so that, in most cases, they can be corrected to prevent a recurrence. There are a few occasions when the solution to an identified or potential problem is very costly in terms of finance and/or resources. The midwifery manager, on behalf of the Trust (or even the Trust Board itself), will need to decide if the risk of not correcting the problem outweighs the costs of correcting it. These are usually rare events, but a Trust view will need to be taken, and so these issues need to be identified and discussed. Managers have a responsibility to their Trust Board to bring such matters to their attention so that a corporate view can be taken, if necessary.

Clinical risk management involves looking at the environment and systems as well as the people, and cannot be undertaken in isolation by one person. There needs to be a culture developed which is built into everyday practice. Clinical risk management needs to be viewed positively to improve client care, and not as a finger-pointing exercise. Collaboration, mutual respect and good communication are vital if effective clinical risk management is to be achieved.

Up until 1997, the manager's responsibility to provide high quality care was implicit. It makes good business sense to ensure that the service provided meets the clients' needs (although it cannot always meet all their demands and expectations) and is of a good quality. Since the National Health Service and Community Care Act 1990 and the introduction of commissioning, health service managers have been required to provide a good quality service as otherwise contracts will be moved to a different provider. Although initially, the emphasis was on effective use of resources, by the middle 1990s commissioners were becoming more interested in quality aspects of care as well as quantity and value for money.

Clinical governance

The White Paper *A First Class Service* (DoH, 1997) laid out the principle of clinical governance, which was later refined in the documents *Clinical Governance – Quality in the New NHS* (DoH, 1999) and *The NHS Plan – A Plan for Investment, A Plan for Reform* (DoH, 2000). Legislation was passed stating that each Trust had a statutory duty to meet the requirements of clinical governance. Trusts were to be accountable for all the care they provided, and Chief Executives and Trust Boards were obliged to ensure the development of local policies.

This was the first time in the history of the NHS that there was a legal requirement to ensure quality of all care provided. The focus was on maintaining consistent, satisfactory and responsive care, and concerns about the quality of care provided were to be at the top of hospital agendas. This meant that midwifery managers had an explicit responsibility to ensure that a cost-effective, evidence-based maternity service was provided. Managers would need to work with all disciplines of healthcare workers as well as supervisors of midwives. Most of the debate around clinical governance concentrated on its effect on the medical profession. Midwifery already had many systems in place that constituted the concept of clinical governance, such as supervision of midwifery, audit, standard setting, consumer participation (Maternity Services Liaison Committees) and evidence-based practice. It was thought that perhaps lessons could be learned in order for clinical governance *per se* to have a positive effect on clinical risk management in maternity service provision. There were an increasing number of general managers who were also heads of midwifery and supervisors of midwives. This placed them in an ideal position to use many of their supervision models and skills when dealing with clinical governance.

The first class service

The White Paper *A First Class Service* (DoH, 1997) stated that National Service frameworks were to be developed over the next 10 years, with clear objectives on the standards of care for each particular service. In order to take these responsibilities forward, managers would need to work with all clinicians. The recommendations from the existing Confidential Enquiries, such as the *Confidential Enquiry into Maternal Deaths*, published annually, have taken many years to be implemented, although the same recommendations recur in each report. How to get clinicians to change practice in the light of evidence continued to be a real dilemma.

Following the First Class Service report, the Commission for Health Improvement (CHI) and The National Institute for Clinical Excellence (NICE) were formed. The core functions for CHI were later refined in *Clinical Governance: Quality in the NHS* (DoH, 1999), and were included in and elaborated on in *The NHS Plan – A Plan for Investment, A Plan for Reform* (DoH 2000). The Commission was charged to ensure the development of the clinical governance process within Trusts, and was to have a key role in providing the public and Secretary of State with the assurance that clinical governance was being implemented appropriately at every level of the NHS. The National Institute for Clinical Excellence was required to set national standards and work to ensure a faster and more uniform uptake of the treatments that work best for patients. The work of both of these groups was to have an impact on maternity services, and the midwifery managers had a responsibility to work closely with all clinicians involved.

Before any new practice is introduced or modified in a unit, there needs to be full evaluation and examination of existing practices. In order for the service to develop to keep pace with new evidence, research, technological advances and client needs, a good working relationship should exist between managers and clinicians. To be effective, managers need to build up good communication with midwives and obstetricians, fostering an environment of collaboration, trust and mutual respect. Most new practices in maternity care involve both medical and midwifery staff, and therefore both disciplines need to work together with the managers and supervisors of midwifery to ensure that both professional groups feel comfortable and competent to change or modify practice.

Many people argued that this environment already existed, but the concept of clinical governance was viewed as new to the medical profession and so increased the risk of fear, resistance and loss of confidence. Most obstetricians and midwives have a very positive working relationship built on support and mutual trust, and it is important that this is not lost. Up until 1999 obstetricians had an *implicit* responsibility to provide a high quality care, but following the new legislation they now have an *explicit* responsibility to demonstrate that their practice is evidence-based and up-to-date. *A First Class Service: Quality in the New NHS* (DoH, 1997) identified the need to make it mandatory for clinicians to take part in the Confidential Enquiries, and this will be monitored as part of the clinical governance process.

Clinical governance could be viewed negatively and, although most midwives and obstetricians already ensure that their practice is up to date and evidence-based, midwifery managers will need to understand the fear that it may cause and work sensitively with clinicians. Clinical risk management will only be effective in an open, collaborative, positive and supportive environment. Any professionals working under the stress of not feeling competent and confident in their practice will not be able to perform to a high standard. This in turn could have a detrimental effect on the standard of care of their colleagues.

The role of the midwifery manager

Midwifery managers are employed by the NHS Trusts to provide a high quality service within existing resources. Management strategy must take account of changing environmental conditions, which not only include research and technological advances but also must include developments in women's needs. Management is largely concerned with managing systems and people. In order to ensure systems are effective, the control loop must be closed by audit/ evaluation on a continual basis. Once shortcomings are identified, corrections need to be put in place and then re-evaluation is essential – 'People are happy to add to the pharmacopoeia; they forget to swallow the medicine' (Beer, 1982).

Clinical risk management is about continually evaluating the current clinical practice and making adjustments where necessary. Many of the adjustments may be more concerned with ensuring that the midwives (and doctors) hold their noses, open their mouths and take the medicine. Much lip service can be paid to proposed changes in practice, but unless the clinicians themselves incorporate the changes into their practices the efforts of risk management will be lost.

It is a statutory responsibility of all midwives to be accountable for their practice (UKCC, 1998), but managers have a responsibility to ensure that midwives are eligible and safe to practise and it is necessary for them to have systems in place. These include the ability to check registration with the UKCC and notification of intention to practise to the local supervisory authority (UKCC, 1998, rule 36), and ensuring that the staff have undertaken all the Trust's statutory training (e.g. annual fire lectures) and comply with all the Trust's policies and procedures.

A manager appoints a midwife to a particular post, and needs to ensure that the midwife is competent to undertake that post at all times. Neither the midwife nor the manager can abdicate their role, and therefore a good working relationship between the two is essential. It is important for managers to ensure that midwives are clear about each of their roles and responsibilities so that confusion or omissions do not arise. Managers cannot hide behind the fact that the midwives are accountable for their own practice, as managers have a responsibility to the Trust who employs them, to ensure eligible, safe and competent practitioners. Likewise, midwives cannot hide behind the fact that they were not reminded to re-register or that problems in their practice were not brought to their attention.

It is a manager's as well as a supervisor of midwives' responsibility to ensure that midwives are aware of and have access to Trust policies and guidelines. There is no point in policies and guidelines being reviewed or introduced if staff are not made aware of their presence. A system must be in place to ensure that this occurs.

Midwives, like all employees, are bound to follow the Trust's policies and procedures, and it is the midwifery manager's responsibility to ensure that they are followed. Midwives must be informed if they breach any policy and procedure, regardless of whether it was detrimental to the mother and baby or not. If necessary, the manager will invoke the Trust's disciplinary procedure. Although disciplinary action is seen as a punitive (and therefore negative) action, it should also be used positively. At the time of the action the midwife must have a clear understanding of what standard is expected in the future, and a timescale set for the standard to be achieved and maintained. A development programme should be planned in conjunction with the supervisor of midwives if there are any breaches of professional rules and codes of practice. Although going through the disciplinary process is extremely stressful, midwives should try to use it constructively. A programme of development at the time could avoid a more serious incident in the future with possibly devastating effects for the midwife and high costs for the Trust. The disciplinary procedure should be viewed as part of the clinical risk management process.

Supervision of midwifery

History of supervision of midwifery

Nearly a century ago, there was a perceived need to regulate midwifery practice. It has now been recognized that this statutory function to regulate midwifery practice should be extended to all clinical practice.

Supervision of midwives is a statutory function, first introduced through the Midwives Act 1902, to ensure that midwifery practice meets the requirements of the Act. Originally most midwives were practising independently or through charities, and the 1902 Act designated local government bodies as local supervising authorities (LSAs). These were established to ensure that midwives complied with the detailed rules of the Central Midwives' Board (CMB) and to receive annual notification of intention to practise from midwives, and were responsible for investigating allegations of professional misconduct by midwives and reporting them to the statutory body. Inspectors of midwives were appointed, but these were not themselves midwives.

It was not until the Midwives Act 1936 that the CMB was empowered to make rules requiring midwives to attend refresher courses, thus recognizing the need to ensure that midwives kept their practice up to date. Medical supervisors were required to be medical officers, and non-medical supervisors were required to be practising midwives but under the control of the medical supervisor, both being employed by the Health Authority. It was this Act that made attendance on a woman in childbirth by an unqualified person illegal.

The Midwives' Code of Practice was not developed until after the Second World War, and then only for England. Northern Ireland and Scotland kept detailed Rules until 1983, when the Nurses, Midwives and Health Visitors Act 1979 was implemented and the United Kingdom Central Council for Nurses, Midwives and Health Visitors (UKCC) was established (it came into effect in 1983).

Current supervision of midwifery

The supervision of midwives continues to evolve rapidly. During the 1990s it became high profile within the context of England's health care, economy and environment. Although it first became a statutory function in 1902, supervision of midwifery is now a recognized and valued role within the midwifery profession, with organizational, legislative and educational structures to underpin it. These are set out in *Midwives' Rules and Code of Practice* (UKCC, 1998).

The purpose of the supervision of midwives is to 'safeguard and enhance the quality of care for the childbearing mother and her family' (ENB, 1996), and therefore needs to be proactive and not reactive. In fulfilling this role, supervision plays a crucial part in developing midwifery practice, and the standards and policies that are developed to ensure safe and high quality of care.

The circumstances in which midwives practise have changed considerably over the years, and whilst supervision continues to focus on the safety of the mother and her baby, the emphasis is now one of supporting professional practice so that childbearing women receive appropriate care working through and with midwives. The benefits that can be achieved for mothers, babies and midwives through good supervision are being recognized, and supervision is being used more positively than ever before to enable and encourage midwives working in the changing maternity services to reflect on, develop and improve their practice.

Supervision of midwifery can be a supportive framework for midwives during the change process. If supervision is used positively, it can empower midwives to identify areas that require change and support them through the change process so that mothers and babies benefit from continually developing practice, and midwives benefit by fulfilling their own potential.

The role of the supervisor of midwives

A supervisor of midwives is appointed by the local supervising authority to exercise supervision over midwives in its geographical area, and must comply with Rule 44 of the *Midwives' Rules and Code of Practice* (UKCC, 1998). This includes the requirement to have successfully completed a programme of preparation, approved by the ENB, prior to taking up the post. Although most supervisors of midwives work for NHS Trusts, it must be remembered that they are directly responsible to the LSA for supervision of midwifery.

The responsibilities of the supervisors are outlined in the *Midwives' Rules and Code of Practice* (UKCC, 1998), and include being an expert practitioner, supervisor, educationalist, researcher and manager. It is important for supervisors of midwives to interact with a variety of people in order to fulfil these roles effectively, and therefore negotiation and communication skills are as important as clinical and managerial skills.

Good clinical practice will reduce clinical risk, and so the responsibility and accountability for clinical practice must be clearly defined and understood by supervisors of midwives, managers and midwives. The areas of responsibility of each person overlap but must be clearly understood so that no confusion, duplication or omissions occur. In contrast to midwifery managers, who manage systems and resources, the focus for a supervisor of midwives is to empower and support midwives so that they can be competent practitioners continually reflecting on and developing their own practice.

It is accepted that management of change for a manager is probably one of the most difficult aspects of the role. A supervisor of midwives needs to have similar expertise in the management of change, and if clinical risk management is to be successful both midwifery managers and supervisors of midwives will need to work together in order to achieve change and so continually develop the maternity service in line with current changes that impact on maternity care.

It has been recognized that people go through the four stages of change to a varying degree, depending on their willingness to see a need for change and the extent to which the change affects themselves. The stages are identified as:

1. Resistance
2. Confusion
3. Integration
4. Commitment.

Part of the role of a supervisor of midwives is to support midwives through this process by encouraging reflective practice. Reflective practice was seen initially as a process of self-criticism, particularly in relation to practice that could have been of a higher standard. Whilst this is true, it should also be used to reflect on good practice and identify why things went well so that this can be replicated. Even with good practice there is often room for further improvement, thus ensuring that midwives stretch themselves and attain their full potential and the service continually develops. Reflection can be a powerful self-motivator, as it teaches practitioners to appraise themselves critically as well as identifying their development. Therefore it should be seen as a valuable process, providing positive feedback as well as being a learning tool. Although reflection is something that most of us do naturally as part of our normal life, reflective practice needs to be encouraged so that it becomes an integral part of clinical practice. It differs from everyday reflection by being documented, referred to and added to over the years. While reflecting and discussing matters with a supervisor, a midwife can identify areas that have potential risk; this then becomes another approach for the management of clinical risk.

Supervisors of midwives should give midwives support as a colleague, counsellor and advisor. This role should be developed in order to promote a positive working relationship, which is conducive to maintaining and improving standards of practice and care (UKCC, 1998, para 34). The *Midwives' Rules and Code of Practice* (UKCC, 1998) clearly states that supervisors of midwives have a responsibility to ensure effective communication between all those determining health service policy and medical staff so that relevant issues are addressed and resolved. This means that supervisors of midwives are required to work with medical staff if care is falling below an acceptable level, irrespective of which professional is responsible. In the past this has entailed education, negotiation and support, but now, with clinical governance, perhaps this aspect of the supervisor of midwives role will be made easier.

Supervisors of midwives have a responsibility to meet at least annually with their supervisees to discuss practice and development needs. This supervision takes the form of an interview, review of records and/or the supervisor working alongside the midwife. This annual review is a proactive approach, not only for the planning of the development of the midwife but also for identifying areas in practice that may be a potential risk. An example of this is record keeping. Reviewing a set of case notes with the midwife is a powerful tool for looking at standards of record keeping and standards of care, as well as creating a climate to discuss philosophies of care. The individual midwife's philosophy of care can have an impact on the way information is provided to the client. This may include stating preferences that may not be evidence-based, so preventing women from making a truly informed choice, as advocated in the *Changing Childbirth* report (DoH, 1993b) and the *Provision of Maternity Services in Scotland: A Policy Review* (Scottish Office, 1993).

Supervisors of midwives also have a role to play in ensuring that all midwives who work on the midwifery bank or through an agency are still eligible to practise. There are regulations regarding the number of hours part-time that midwives must work in order to be eligible to notify their intention to practise, but it is important that these midwives keep themselves up to date. For those midwives who only work occasionally, it is important that they are aware of the need to ensure that their practice is safe and evidence-based. It is especially important for these midwives to meet with their named supervisors of midwives so as to plan a programme of development that will ensure that they not only fulfil their professional requirements for registration but also that they are confident and competent to practise.

It is in the Trust's interests to ensure that all their employees are safe to practise and aware of all policies and procedures. It is not uncommon for non-permanent staff to be involved in litigation cases because of a breakdown of communication, or through unfamiliarity with Trust policies. Therefore it is essential for supervisors of midwives to ensure that all midwives, regardless of the number of hours worked, are competent, safe practitioners who are familiar with local policies, procedures and guidelines. Midwifery managers will be trying to ensure that non-permanent staff usage is kept to the minimum, although, because of the national shortage of midwives, this is frequently very difficult if not impossible.

Supervisors of midwives also have a responsibility to ensure effective communication links between themselves and those determining health service policy, and a responsibility to ensure that they are involved in the formulation and review of policies and guidelines relating to maternity care. As has been stated earlier in the chapter, all maternity practice impinges on midwives, who have a responsibility to be the woman's advocate. Therefore midwives must understand the rationale behind policies and guidelines if they are to give full, unbiased information so that the woman and her partner can make informed choices. Following on from being involved in their formulation, it is also a supervisor's responsibility to ensure that midwives are made aware of new and updated policies, procedures and guidelines.

The role of the supervisor of midwives in clinical risk management

As the aim of clinical risk management is to improve the quality of care, supervisors of midwives have a duty to become involved in risk management and clinical audit if they are to fulfil their function to ensure safety for mothers and babies.

It has already been shown that practitioners must be able to see the need to change their own practice rather than just be instructed to do so. Midwives have a duty to ensure their practice is up to date; therefore supervisors need to work with midwives, encouraging reflective practice so that care is continually evaluated and updated and change in practice is sustained. Strategies for reducing and eliminating clinical risk can only be effective if they are sustainable. It is a waste of everyone's time to alter the way care is delivered, only to find in a few months time that old practices have crept back. One of the fundamental principles for managing change is that change can only be managed effectively if the practitioners themselves recognize the need for change and have the skills and confidence to carry it out.

Midwives are authorized by law to carry full responsibility for the care of childbearing women throughout pregnancy, labour, delivery and the puerperium without recourse to a doctor, unless there is a deviation from the norm. It is crucial that midwives are competent to carry out this responsibility, and are able to maintain and develop their competence (ENB, 1997). Supervisors can help midwives to achieve this through their role as colleague, counsellor and advisor.

The midwife's role in clinical risk management

The *Midwives' Rules and Code of Practice* (UKCC, 1998, p. 25) states:

> *Each midwife as a practitioner of midwifery is accountable for her or his own practice in whatever environment s/he practises. The standard of practice in the delivery of midwifery care shall be that which is acceptable in the context of current knowledge and clinical developments. In all*

circumstances the safety and welfare of the mother and her baby must be of primary importance.

As a practising midwife, you are accountable for your own practice in whatever environment you are practising. In all circumstances, the safety and welfare of the mother and her baby are of primary importance.

The Nurses, Midwives and Health Visitors Act 1979 and the amending act of 1992 provided a framework for the development of the UKCC's policy documents, such as *Midwives' Rules and Code of Practice* (UKCC, 1998). Such legislation affects the boundaries for midwifery practice and working arrangements, and the future development of the midwifery profession. In the *Code of Professional Conduct* (UKCC, 1992) professional accountability is clearly identified. Midwives have a statutory duty to ensure that they 'maintain and improve their professional knowledge and competence' and 'acknowledge any limitations' in these areas. Midwives must decline to undertake any duties or responsibilities unless they are competent and confident to do so in a safe and skilled manner.

This responsibility was highlighted during the introduction of water births. Considerable pressure can be exerted on midwives if they are not proficient to conduct a water birth and a client is requesting one. Many midwives have felt pressurized by clients to provide care through a water birth because they are known to the client, yet they have not acquired an acceptable skill in this particular field. Another dilemma posed is if the midwife is the only member of the team who has this skill but does not wish to cover the impending delivery on a 24-hour on-call basis. In order to manage the clinical risk midwives and supervisors need to work together to resolve the issues, meeting the client's and the midwife's needs. The midwife has a responsibility to discuss such situations with the named supervisor of midwives as soon as they become apparent. In the former situation a supervisor could arrange for a colleague, skilled in water births, to conduct the delivery, with the named midwife supporting the client whilst learning the skill at the same time. In the latter case, the supervisor could arrange with the manager for a team of midwives who have skills in water births to meet and if possible care for the woman antenatally so that a midwife known to the woman can conduct the delivery. Because of the very nature of the supervisor of midwives' role, the midwives who have that particular skill will be known or accessible. The supervisor can and invariably does meet with the mother, explaining the risks involved in midwives working too many hours and becoming tired, whilst also explaining the midwives' professional responsibilities to be competent and safe to practise and not undertake a practice in which they have not received sufficient training. This has proved helpful in ensuring that a good relationship between midwife and client is maintained.

Some problems have arisen regarding Trust policies for water births. Supervisors of midwives need to ensure that, in order for a midwife to comply with Trust policies, they do not have to contravene their professional codes of practice. Midwives have a statutory duty to attend a woman in labour. If a Trust policy states that a woman must leave the water for the birth of her baby and/or the delivery of the placenta and membranes and the woman refuses, the midwife would contravene the *Midwives' Code of Practice* if she refused to attend the woman or physically tried to remove her from the water. A well-known case in

East Hertfordshire (Carlisle, 1994) highlighted the dilemmas that midwives could face.

Midwives have a statutory responsibility to work with supervisors of midwives in order for problems to be shared and a resolution achieved before a conflict situation arises, as both have an explicit responsibility to provide optimum care for mothers and babies (UKCC, 1998, p. 33/34 para 34).

Identifying clinical risk situations

As stated previously, it is important that potential clinical risk situations are identified as soon as possible. It is not enough to look only at situations that have already occurred. Time, effort and money will be saved if the management of clinical risk is proactive. Of course, any identified clinical risk situation needs to be identified and investigated, and a strategy formulated to ensure that it does not recur. Most NHS Trusts have reporting mechanisms in place to identify untoward incidents. Many Trusts go further by encouraging identification of 'near misses' or potential risks. For example, a piece of equipment breaking down is a potential risk if there are not sufficient resources to replace it while it is being repaired. The same can be true if a policy is not followed, even if the clinical outcome is good, because the next time this may not be the case. In the latter instance the policy will need to be reviewed to ensure that it is still appropriate and to identify any training issues that need to be addressed.

Clinical risk situations are best identified by a multi-professional team, so that all aspects are considered. As professionals all have codes of practice within which to work, it is essential that policies and guidelines are not formulated that will necessitate one or more professionals having to work outside their rules and codes of practice.

A risk management group

The risk management group is a powerful tool and should be seen as avoiding litigation, not evading it (Clements, 1992). When looking at organizations, problems that seem to be resistant to solutions may be identified. It has been found that rather than keep trying to impose solutions it is better to pose the problem in a new and solvable way (Beer, 1966). The same can be true for clinical risk problems. The most effective risk management groups are multi-disciplinary and multi-professional. Even when looking at clinical risk as a purely midwifery-related issue it is important to obtain the medical view. Both midwives and medical personnel need to work as a team, and a different professional's view may offer a different perspective, thus posing the problem in a new and solvable way. Each group should have senior obstetric, senior midwifery and legal input, with paediatric and anaesthetic representation as necessary. The numbers from each discipline will depend on the size of the unit. The senior midwifery representation should include a supervisor of midwives.

It is to the benefit of the client that both midwifery managers and supervisors of midwives work closely together in developing a risk management group, but one co-ordinator with either midwifery or medical knowledge should be appointed. The manager has a specific responsibility to reduce the risk of litigation, and the supervisor has a specific statutory responsibility to ensure the safety of mothers and babies. Both have a responsibility to ensure that a high quality service is provided, and therefore both have an interest in an effective risk management group.

For clinical risk management to be effective there needs to be a list of conditions where a risk factor may be present, and common examples include the following.

Neonatal conditions:

- An Apgar score of 4 or less
- A baby unexpectedly admitted to the neonatal unit
- Intrapartum stillbirth
- Undiagnosed abnormality
- Delay/difficulty with paediatric resuscitation
- Birth trauma to the baby during delivery
- Breaches of infant security.

Maternal conditions:

- Maternal death
- Unexpected deterioration in the mother's condition
- Eclamptic fit or collapse
- Serious soft tissue injury (e.g. a third-degree tear, a ruptured uterus or a bladder injury)
- Postpartum haemorrhage
- Undiagnosed breech presentation at delivery.

Once an agreed condition occurs the case is referred to the group's co-ordinator, who will review the case or arrange for another member of the group to do so. It is usually necessary to have discussions with the relevant staff, and a summary written for presentation to the group. The group can then decide if written statements would be prudent even if the question of litigation has not been raised. Comprehensive records or statements made soon after an incident are more likely to be accurate, and will assist staff in recalling events if required to do so at a later stage (Symon, 1997).

Setting standards of practice and care

In order for the risk management group to be effective, members of the group need to ensure that standards of care are set. It is the responsibility of managers and supervisors to ensure that the maternity department's strategy fits in with the overall quality of care audit strategy for the Trust.

A proactive part of the risk management process is to recognize where quality of care can be improved, without waiting for a problem to arise. However, before identifying improvements an accepted standard of care must be set against which comparisons can be made. Standards of care pertaining to midwifery and maternity care should be set by a cross-section of the clinicians involved. For example, standards for record keeping, which involve doctors as well as mid-wives, need to be agreed by both disciplines, whereas standards for advice on breast feeding need to involve health visitors and neonatal nurses as well as midwives, thus aiming to ensure continuity of care and advice. Auditing standards on a regular basis contributes to the risk management process. Care that falls short of the agreed standards can be identified before a condition that has been identified as a potential risk occurs – an example of this would be a midwife not using an agreed suture material and/or technique for perineal suturing. In some instances agreed timescales need to be included so that a plan can be developed in order to achieve an acceptable level. Standards of care must be realistic and achievable, and if there is a large gap between acceptable standards and current practice a timescale will help professionals to work towards the goal without feeling demoralized and demotivated. If the latter occurs, the standard will never be achieved.

Clinical audit

Audit of clinical practice is an essential part of clinical risk management. It is essential that, like the control loop, the audit cycle of the standards of practice and care is completed with evaluation, and that the process is reiterative. Again, supervisors of midwives and managers have found that setting up working groups consisting of all grades of medical and midwifery staff has been useful in auditing standards. It is essential that an agreed checklist is used at each audit so that objective comparisons can be made and progress assessed. In order to create a positive environment where results of audits can be presented publicly and lessons learned, the reports of individual practice should be anonymized. However, it will be the supervisor's and manager's responsibility to discuss specific practice issues with individuals if it becomes apparent during the auditing process that there is a particular training need.

Reviews of stillbirths and early neonatal deaths

Many Trusts have regular meetings to review all the stillbirths and early neonatal deaths in the unit. The most constructive and effective meetings are attended by all grades of obstetricians, paediatricians/neonatologists, midwives and paediatric/neonatal nurses, GPs, and, where possible, a pathologist and a pharmacist. For benefits to be gained, the climate needs to be honest, open, supportive and constructive. It is extremely valuable to have care discussed from all the professionals' viewpoints. In some cases, the care provided by the obstetrician may have a direct bearing on the care provided by the neonatologist – such an example is drugs given in labour, which may have a positive or adverse affect on the outcome for the baby. These issues need to be discussed. In many cases the outcome may not be affected, but that does not mean that the care provided could not have been improved.

Managers have a responsibility to facilitate midwives' attendance at these meetings, especially those midwives involved in the cases that are to be discussed.

Supervisors of midwives have a dual role at the meetings. Primarily they are concerned about the standard of care provided, but they can also provide support to midwives who may feel intimidated in challenging a medical viewpoint or anxious if the case has involved them. Some clinicians can feel threatened discussing a case in an open forum in case substandard care is identified. It is important that the meetings are not fault finding but constructive. If handled properly, these meetings are a good learning experience for all who attend. It must be accepted that it is difficult to arrange a time that is mutually suitable for so many clinicians with different commitments, but it is a valuable contribution to clinical risk management and therefore every effort ought to be made.

Debriefing following childbirth service

Debriefing following childbirth has been used positively for a risk management cycle (Dineen, 1996; Smith and Mitchell, 1996). During childbirth women and their partners are often in an anxious state, in pain, and have difficulty understanding or remembering information given. Debriefing discussions following childbirth can be extremely helpful in explaining why a particular course of action was taken, and given at a time when the mother is more likely to understand and remember. It has also been found to be valuable in informing clinicians how their care has been *perceived* by the client. Debriefing discussions not only help to reduce the risk of psychological problems or post-traumatic syndrome (American Psychiatric Association, 1994) but have also been found to reduce the number of complaints, as women are able to understand the rationale for management whilst being given the opportunity to explain their views and perceptions of care. This aids good communication. The perception of the recipient often varies from that of the giver. In the words of the immortal bard Robert Burns: 'O wad some Pow'r the giftie gie us to see ourselves as others see us!' (Burns, 1784).

The debriefing team needs to be supported by a manager and supervisor of midwives so that the women's comments can be used positively to improve the quality of care. The team and the women themselves need to be very clear that it is not a counselling service, nor an official complaints procedure, and that it is for discussing and explaining the care with no personal views being stated by the midwives. Should the midwives identify that more in-depth counselling is required, the woman must be referred to the appropriate agency. If it becomes evident that the woman wishes to lodge a formal complaint, the complaints procedure must be explained, written information of the procedure given and, if required, arrangements made for a manager to meet with the complainant. As it is not a counselling service the midwives involved will not need formal counselling for themselves, but it has been found to be helpful to meet with a supervisor of midwives individually and as a group. These interviews will be confidential, but if a name keeps recurring it will be necessary for the supervisor to meet with the individual identified and together to plan a way forward and/or address any training needs. In the author's local project, the recurring theme from the debriefing sessions is that the mothers and their partners feel that there has been a lack of effective communication.

Effective use of resources

Three main recurring themes during the clinical risk management process are record keeping, communication and staffing issues. At first glance it may be thought that the latter comes only within the midwifery manager's remit, but it must been seen as an important issue for consideration by the supervisor of midwives as well as by the midwives themselves. When staffing issues are identified, the way in which staff resources have been allocated and utilized will need to be considered, as obtaining additional staff is not always possible and may not always solve the problem. This highlights the need for managers, supervisors and midwives to work together to look at best practice. As practice is continually developing and the demarcation between the roles of midwives and doctors becomes more blurred, it is essential to ensure that outdated and/or non-evidence-based practices are not continued when new practices have been introduced to replace them. It is easy in a very busy work schedule to introduce new practices without assessing the impact on existing ones and considering the need to cease some in order to avoid duplication. Duplication of care can be very confusing for the client, does not enhance care, and is a waste of resources. There is a national shortage of midwives, so it is essential that midwives utilize their time effectively.

Continuity of care and carer has been discussed at length in many venues since the publication of *Changing Childbirth* (DoH, 1993b). There has long been the expectation that:

- Every mother will deliver a perfect baby
- Pregnancy is a happy and normal life event
- Motherhood will be synonymous with love and nurturing
- Professionals will be supportive, knowledgeable and safe practitioners.

Now there is another expectation added to these: that there will be continuity of care and carer. A criticism levied at healthcare professionals is that of conflicting advice. If the number of professionals involved in the care of a woman is reduced, the likelihood of conflicting advice and change in care plans will be reduced. Since the introduction of caseload and small-team midwifery many hospitals have noticed a reduction in the number of complaints, as the women are more satisfied with this type of care when compared to traditional care (Hodnett, 1998). However, issues regarding midwife burnout are now beginning to be identified (Sandall, 1997).

Supervisors and managers have a joint responsibility to work with midwives to look at models of care that can reduce the number of professionals involved in a woman's care and ensure that, even when continuity of carer is not achieved, the care and advice offered is consistent. Continuity of carer and care is good practice whilst being more cost effective and reducing complaints. However, as highlighted previously, a sensible balance must be achieved to ensure that midwives are not becoming overtired in order to provide continuity of carer.

Professional development for midwives

In order to ensure a high quality, safe maternity service, it is essential that midwives' practice is based on current evidence and research and is centred on women's needs. Midwives have an accountability to ensure that their clinical practice and knowledge are up to date. Supervisors of midwives have a responsibility to work with midwives, helping them to identify development needs and supporting them through professional development. Professional development does not just mean attendance at study days and courses, but there is a real need to look at various forms of development. Shadowing colleagues, working in different areas within and outside Trust settings, reading, reflecting on practice, participation in standard setting, audit groups and workshops are among many methods that need to be considered. No one method will be appropriate for all midwives, and just as individualized care is planned for a woman, so too is there a need to plan professional development for individual midwives on an ongoing basis.

Whilst midwives and supervisors of midwives are responsible for identifying training and development needs, the midwifery managers have a responsibility to work with staff and facilitate development opportunities. Training and professional development must be taken seriously and included in any service's business plan if clinical risk management is to be effective. Highly skilled, competent and up-to-date practitioners are more likely to provide safe, high quality care, which in turn will reduce clinical risk. Like management of clinical risk, training and development needs to be an integral part of the maternity service and the responsibility shared by midwives, midwifery managers and supervisors of midwives alike.

Conclusion

Supervisors of midwives, managers, midwives and clients all play an important part in clinical risk management. This chapter has examined the roles and responsibilities of the professionals in this process. It has also emphasized the value of positive relationships between professionals, and with clients, in managing clinical risk effectively.

Systems and processes need to be in place that will ensure effective management of clinical risk. Management concentrates on the effective use of resources to provide a quality maternity service, and on the systems, whereas the prime focus of supervision is to ensure that a high standard of care is provided by empowering midwives.

The environment in which midwifery care is provided has been greatly affected by increasing technology, emerging evidence, increasing research, and women's needs. The concept of supervision was first introduced by legislation in 1902, but the tools of supervision were developed by later legislation that introduced rules, codes of practice and educational requirements. Although the focus remains on the safety of mother and her baby, it has developed so that it concentrates on empowering midwives instead of being a punitive function.

Midwifery management has also developed, recognizing the need to manage clinical risk positively and to improve the maternity service by trying to put the client needs at the centre of service provision.

An honest and open climate, which is supportive of all clinicians, must exist so that practice can be evaluated and developed without demoralizing and destroying professional confidence. Managers, supervisors and midwives must work closely together, accepting joint responsibility for continually identifying risk and potential risk situations. Complaints and other identified risk situations should be viewed positively, and whatever the medicine, it should be swallowed.

Clinical risk management systems are a joint responsibility for all clinicians, managers and supervisors of midwives, both individually and collectively, and must be reiterative processes. Healthcare teams cannot be complacent, but must be forever seeking to improve practice and to build on their own professional development.

Midwifery managers and supervisors must continue to work closely together in order to manage clinical risk to the greatest benefit of mothers, babies and midwives.

References

American Psychiatric Association (1994). *Diagnostic and Statistical Manual of Mental Disorders*, 4th edn (DSM-IV). American Psychiatric Association.

Beer, S. (1982). The Lindsey Sutcliffe Memorial Lecture.

Beer, S. (1996). *Decision and Control*. John Wiley & Sons.

Burns, R. (1784). To a Louse, On seeing one on a Bonnet at Church.

Carlisle, D. (1994). A mother's right to choose? *Nursing Times*, **90(13)**, 14–15.

Clements, R. V. (1992). Defensive medicine – is this where risk management leads? *Health Service J.*, **Apr**.

Collins New English Dictionary (1997). HarperCollins.

Department of Health (1993a). *Risk Management in the NHS*. HMSO.

Department of Health (1993b) *Changing Childbirth: Report of the Expert Maternity Group*. HMSO

Department of Health (1997). *A First Class Service: Quality in the New NHS*. HMSO.

Department of Health (1999). *Clinical Governance – Quality in the New NHS*. HMSO.

Department of Health (2000). *The NHS Plan – A Plan for Investment, A Plan for Reform*. HMSO.

Dineen, M. (1996). Clinical risk management – a pragmatic approach. *Br. J. Midwifery*, **4(8)** (Suppl.).

English National Board for Nursing, Midwifery and Health Visiting (1996). *Supervision of Midwives: The English National Board's Guidance to Local Supervising Authorities and Supervisors of Midwives*, p. 13. ENB.

English National Board for Nursing, Midwifery and Health Visiting (1997). *Module 1, Preparation of Supervisors of Midwives: Supervision and You: What is Your Role?*, p.11 para.1.1. ENB.

Hodnett, E. D. (1998). Continuity of Caregivers during Pregnancy and Childbirth. *Cochrane Review*, in the Cochrane Library Issue 4. Update Software.

Sandall, J. (1997). Midwives' burnout and continuity of care. *Br. J. Midwifery*, **5(2)**, 106–11.

Scottish Office (Home and Health Department) (1993). *Provision of Maternity Services in Scotland: A Policy Review*. HMSO.

Smith, J. and Mitchell, S. (1996). Debriefing after childbirth – a tool for effective risk management. *Br. J. Midwifery*, **4(8)** (Suppl.).

Symon, A. (1997). Midwives and litigation: allegations of clinical errors. *Br. J. Midwifery*, **5(1)**, 17–19.

United Kingdom Central Council for Nursing, Midwifery and Health Visiting (1992). *Code of Professional Conduct*. UKCC.

United Kingdom Central Council for Nursing, Midwifery and Health Visiting (1993). *Midwives' Rules*. UKCC.

United Kingdom Central Council for Nursing, Midwifery and Health Visiting (1994). *Midwives' Code of Practice*. UKCC.

United Kingdom Central Council for Nursing, Midwifery and Health Visiting (1998). *Midwives' Rules and Code of Practice*. UKCC.

6

Consent issues during pregnancy and childbirth

Liz Rodgers

Introduction

The fact that medical treatment should not be given to a patient unless he or she consents is a concept familiar to all healthcare workers. Midwives, by virtue of their close involvement with a patient, play a crucial role where the patient's consent to treatment is an issue. An understanding of the legal concept of consent, and the problem areas within the concept, is essential for all practising midwives. In this chapter, therefore, the legal meaning of consent is outlined, together with the law's response to the less routine cases of childbirth.

Throughout the chapter the word treatment is taken to refer to any medical intervention necessary during pregnancy and birth. It is acknowledged, however, that pregnancy is not an illness, and hence treatment is at times an inappropriate term to apply.

The meaning of consent

Patient autonomy

The starting point for the legal doctrine of consent is one of patient autonomy – the right of self-rule and determination. The principle is commonly cited thus (*per* Cardozo J, in Schloendorff *v.* Society of New York Hospital [1914]):

> *Every human being of adult years and sound mind has the right to determine what shall be done with his own body.*

Implicit within this statement is the idea that, just as treatment can be agreed to, an adult patient of sound mind has a right to refuse treatment that is proposed. It is in these situations that the courts may be asked to intervene. That court actions arise as a result of a patient's refusal is not surprising – the patient's refusal may be seen as irrational and certainly not in his or her best interests by the healthcare team, and refusal does not sit easily with the medical profession's perceived duty to its patients. However, a failure to agree with the patient's refusal does not automatically permit the medical team to override that decision:

> *A man or woman of full age and sound understanding may choose to reject medical advice and medical ... treatment whether partially or in its entirety. A decision to refuse medical treatment by a patient*

capable of making the decision does not have to be sensible, rational or well-considered.

> (*per* Butler-Sloss LJ in *re* T (adult: refusal of treatment) [1992])

What is important, therefore, is an appreciation by midwives of when their patients will be of 'full age and sound understanding' and hence able to make treatment decisions and treatment refusals.

Full age

A patient is of full age once the age of majority has been reached. In England, this is currently set at 18 years. However, due to the impact of statute and case law within the area of children's rights, there exist some situations where an individual who is below the age of 18 can consent to (or refuse) medical treatment. The legal rules surrounding pregnant young adults will be considered later.

Sound understanding

Before patients are deemed legally able to make treatment decisions, they must satisfy three tests that go to make up the notion of sound understanding. Whilst it is ultimately for a court to decide these issues in disputed cases, practitioners must also be well versed in the application of the tests and will be relied upon to give testimony in the event of an application to court.

Stage 1: does the patient have capacity to consent?

Capacity in this regard refers to the ability of the patient to understand the nature of treatment decisions and to make a choice based on the information provided. In *re* C (Adult: refusal of treatment) [1994], the legal steps to establish a patient's understanding were set out. Thorpe J formulated these steps as follows:

> *first, comprehending and retaining treatment information, second, believing it and, third, weighing it in the balance to arrive at choice.*

These steps have been incorporated into two subsequent cases dealing with pregnant patients who were deemed to need Caesarean sections. In Norfolk and Norwich Healthcare (NHS) Trust *v.* W [1996], the consultant psychiatrist was asked three questions in relation to the patient:

1. Is she capable of comprehending and retaining information about the proposed treatment?
2. Is she capable of believing the information given to her about her treatment?
3. Is she capable of weighing such information in the balance to make a choice?

This format of questioning to ascertain capacity was also applied in Tameside and Glossop Acute Services Trust *v.* CH [1996], and is an approach that would be suitable for adoption by any midwife discussing treatment decisions with a patient. Only if the questions can be answered in the affirmative will the patient be deemed to be capable. It would be all too easy to interpret the irrational choice of a patient at the third question as being a sign that the patient is not in fact weighing up the pros and cons of the treatment options to arrive at a decision. In the area of pregnancy this is all too likely, since an irrational choice that may result in harm to the fetus would for many seem to fall short of true capacity. In the case of *re* MB [1997], the judge concluded:

> *A competent woman who has the capacity to decide may ... choose not to have medical intervention, even though the consequence may be the death or serious handicap of the child she bears, or her own death. In that event the courts do not have the jurisdiction to declare medical intervention lawful.*

This clearly indicates the rights of patients to determine their own fate, and that of any fetus, if they can be deemed capable. The added difficulty with this proposition is the need for the degree of seriousness of decision-making to be compatible with the degree of capacity. In *re* T (Adult: refusal of medical treatment) [1992], the medical practitioners were, according to Lord Donaldson, to:

> *... consider whether at {the} time {of making the decision} he had a capacity which was commensurate with the gravity of the decision which he purported to make. The more serious the decision, the greater the capacity required.*

This view was supported in the case of *re* MB. As to the rights of the fetus, it should be noted that the courts will not accord 'rights' to the unborn fetus, and it is currently accepted law that a fetus has no right to life:

> *Throughout this judgement I have referred to 'the fetus' because I wish to emphasize that the focus of my judicial attention was upon the interests of the patient herself, and not upon the interests of the fetus which she bore.*
>
> (*per* Johnson J. in Norfolk and Norwich Healthcare NHS Trust *v.* W [1996])

For a further discussion, see cases such as *re* F (In utero) [1988] (referred to in Tameside), which overturned the comments made by the judge in *re* S (Adult: refusal of medical treatment) [1993]. Full citations are given at the end of this chapter. The father of the child may also be perceived as having rights, and this issue will be considered later.

Stage 2: consent must be given free from duress

For any consent to treatment to be valid it must be given freely, without any form of coercion being applied to the patient. The legal basis for this require-ment is that the patient must be making the decision him/herself, and not, according to Lord Donaldson in *re* T (Adult: refusal of treatment) [1992]:

> *... merely saying it for a quiet life, to satisfy someone else or because the advice and persuasion to which he had been subjected is such that he can no longer think and decide for himself.*

Persuasion can come from a variety of sources, and professionals involved must be aware that they themselves may act in a manner that influences a patient's choice. Indeed, it is hard to establish where professional guidance becomes so influential that the patient's ability to choose has disappeared, and any disputed cases would be judged on their facts.

Stage 3: is the patient suitably informed?

Linked to the first stage (capacity to consent), the patient must be suitably informed before any treatment decisions can be classed as valid. The law in the UK does not require 'informed consent' as it is practised in the USA. Patients do not have to be told of all the risks and facts related to their treatment options; they merely have to be told enough to enable them to make a choice that links in to the final aspect of the understanding test outlined above. Any failure to provide patients with sufficient information to make a choice in itself may not vitiate consent, although this may be actionable in negligence. Misinforming a patient as to the treatment risks or the deliberate withholding of information may, however, result in the patient's consent being invalid.

Consequences for treating in the absence of consent

If a patient is treated in the absence of consent the medical practitioner may be liable in negligence for damages, since failure to ensure that consent is real can constitute a breach of the duty of care owed by a practitioner to the patient. In addition, the patient may utilize the tortious action of battery. To establish this civil wrong, the patient needs to prove that the defendant (the practitioner) touched them in a harmful or offensive manner without the giving of consent and without lawful justification. The fact that a practitioner is acting in a way designed ultimately to promote the wellbeing of the patient is irrelevant. This is due to the interpretation of touching another without consent as being a harmful act in itself. If civil action is pursued, the remedy granted in the event of success would be financial compensation.

When the patient cannot consent

If a patient cannot consent, or is deemed incapable of consenting after the application of the above principles, again the law can be looked to by way of assistance. In many cases inability to consent will arise through unconsciousness – perhaps as a result of a road traffic accident or coma, or as a consequence of an existing illness, whether physical or mental. In these situations the law will permit treatment in the absence of consent:

> ... *the practitioner can lawfully treat the patient in accordance with his clinical judgement of what is in the patient's best interests.*
>
> (*per* Lord Donaldson in *re* T (Adult: refusal of treatment) [1992])

What is in a patient's best interests will to a certain extent depend upon the individual facts of the case and the medical evidence available. However, there are fundamental elements to the decision:

> *The operation or other treatment will be in their best interests if, but only if, it is carried out in order either to save their lives or to ensure improvement or to prevent deterioration in their physical or mental health.*
>
> (*per* Lord Brandon in *re* F (In utero) [1988])

In the case of Airedale NHS Trust *v.* Bland [1993], the judge (Lord Goff) noted that:

> *... medical treatment or care may be provided for a number of different purposes. It may be provided for example as an aid to diagnosis, for the treatment of physical or mental injury or illness, to alleviate pain or distress ... But for my part I cannot see that medical treatment is appropriate ... simply to prolong a patient's life when such treatment has no therapeutic purpose of any kind.*

From these extracts the need for treatment to be of a therapeutic benefit, but also to be the least intervention necessary at the time of treating the patient, should be clear. The assessment of what treatment will in fact be in the patient's best interests will normally rest with the medical team, with the court being called in to adjudicate in the event of disagreement. Whilst it is not obligatory for the medical team to consult with the incapable patient's relatives, this is something that is commonly done. The relatives' wishes should never be seen as the overriding factor, and nor should relatives be permitted to give consent to treatment for any adult patient:

> *There seems to be a view in the medical profession that in such emergency circumstances the next of kin should be asked to consent on behalf of the patient and that, if possible, treatment should be postponed until that consent has been obtained. This is a misconception because the next of kin has no legal rights either to consent or to refuse consent.*
>
> (*per* Lord Donaldson in *re* T (Adult: refusal of treatment [1992])

Indeed, whilst the courts may be asked to adjudicate, they too have no powers to consent – the court's role is merely to determine whether treatment is legal. The same principles of law apply equally to those patients who are incapable of making a decision, whether the cause is temporary or permanent.

Application of the principle

The unconscious pregnant woman

Insofar as treatment is directed towards the patient herself, and is for a therapeutic purpose, there are generally no difficulties in applying the 'best interests' test. Problems may arise where the patient is unconscious, with a poor prognosis, or even being maintained by virtue of mechanical means. In this situation, the question must be whether it is legally permissible to continue to prolong life merely to permit the fetus to mature to full term, or mature sufficiently to be viable. That this has happened is certain (see, for example, Mail Newspapers PLC *v.* Express Newspapers PLC [1987]), and for many this would be seen as the correct approach to a patient's care. In 1993, a British Medical Association spokesperson went on record as saying:

> *If the pregnancy had run for 26–27 weeks it would be uncontroversial to maintain the mother on a life support system to give her baby the best chance of survival.*
>
> (*The Telegraph*, 18 January 1993).

However, this assumption may be made on the basis of moral and ethical principles rather than purely legal ones. If the patient's life is prolonged merely in order to enable induced birth at some future point in time, it is necessary to consider the legal basis for so doing. It could be suggested that permitting the unconscious patient to carry the fetus to term is in the patient's (the woman's) best interests. Alternatively, it could be suggested that it is in the interests of the fetus, or even that it is in the interests of the father to do so. In all three of these possibilities there arise difficult legal arguments.

Starting with the 'best interests' of the patient, on first glance this appears to be supported by the principles of treatment in an emergency expounded in the case of *re* F (In utero) [1988]. However, on careful analysis it is questionable whether there is legal validity for this course of action. Can it really be said that maintaining a patient who but for the artificial means of sustaining breathing etc. would otherwise die or be declared brain dead, is therapeutic treatment? In what way does the treatment save life (other than that of the fetus) or prevent a deterioration of the woman's condition? In addition, can it really be argued that a patient in a persistent vegetative state (PVS), or who is being ventilated mechanically, has any best interests? This was a point raised by Lord Mustill in the Airedale NHS Trust *v.* Bland [1993] case. Clearly here the worst-case scenario is being considered, but it is necessary to do so to highlight the potential conflicts between ethical or moral practice and legal rules.

Looking at the alternative arguments, the rights of the fetus have already been touched upon. In law it is clear that a fetus has no right to life, and hence treating the patient to preserve the life of the fetus is, in legal terms, inherently wrong. In addition, the question of when this course of action would be commenced must be raised. Would it be right to distinguish between a woman who has conceived merely 2 weeks previously and one who is nearly at full term?

If the existence of a fetus that could survive to viability cannot provide legal validity for continuing to maintain the woman patient, the ability of the father to do so needs addressing. Again, from the earlier comments, the answer to this issue should be apparent – a father has no legal rights to insist upon or agree to the woman remaining on support systems. Analogies from case law can be made with regard to the legal rights of a father to prevent the woman obtaining an abortion. In two cases in England and Wales this question has been considered, with the same result. In Paton *v.* Trustees of British Pregnancy Advisory Service [1978], a husband sought an injunction to prevent his wife from terminating her pregnancy. The court stated (*per* Sir George Baker):

> *The 1967 [Abortion] Act gives no right to a father to be consulted in respect of the termination of a pregnancy ... The husband, therefore, in my view, has no legal right enforceable at law or in equity to stop his wife having this abortion or to stop the doctors from carrying out the abortion.*

In C *v.* S [1987] a similar situation arose, although in this case the father was not married to the mother. In this case he tried to prevent the abortion by claiming that the doctors would be breaching the Infant Life (Preservation) Act 1929. Again the action failed – the court did not agree that the fetus was viable and also felt that the putative father did not have any status, or right, to bring the action to prevent the abortion.

The analogy with continuing a pregnancy is clear, and if the matter were to be pursued through the courts it is likely (although not certain) that the courts would follow the existing principle of not giving rights to the father to dictate treatment choices.

The mentally incapable pregnant woman

Where a woman is unable to make a decision due to her incapacity, the best interests test will still apply unless the patient is suffering from a defined mental illness, which may enable the patient to be treated under the provisions of the Mental Health Act 1983. The relationship between this latter Act and non-consenting pregnant patients is one that has recently come to the fore, and throughout the mid-1990s several cases were dealt with by the courts where the 1983 Act was argued to be relevant.

Under the Mental Health Act 1983, a patient who is suffering from a defined mental illness and who is formally detained in hospital under the Act may in certain situations be treated without his or her consent being needed. Section 63 of the Act outlines the normal situations where non-consensual treatment can be given – the treatment must be for the mental illness, and treatment can only last for a total of 3 months. Whilst treatment related to pregnancy naturally can extend beyond 3 months, the question of treatment being for the mental illness is more pertinent. In the Tameside case, the patient suffered from paranoid schizophrenia and had been formally detained under the 1983 legislation. The obstetrician planned to induce labour due to intrauterine growth retardation of the fetus, but was aware that the patient was apt to resist treatment. Given the possible need to carry out a Caesarean section, authority to conduct the relevant procedure, if necessary, was sought. Whilst the judge found that the patient was unable to consent due to her incapacity, he did not make a declaration authorizing treatment under the common law powers of treating in the patient's best interests, as restraint of the patient may have been needed. Instead, the declaration was granted under the Mental Health Act 1983 (*per* Wall J, Tameside and Glossop Acute Services Trust *v.* CH [1996]):

> *Is the question of inducing the defendant's labour and/or causing her to be delivered of her child by Caesarean section 'entirely unconnected' with her mental disorder? At first blush, it might appear difficult to say that performance of a Caesarean section is medical treatment for the defendant's mental disorder: ... on the facts of this case so to hold would be 'too atomistic a view' ... There are several strands ... which ... bring the proposed treatment within section 63 of the Act. First, there is the proposition that an ancillary reason for the induction and, if necessary, the birth by Caesarean section is to prevent a deterioration in the defendant's mental state. Secondly, there is ... evidence ... that in order for the treatment of her schizophrenia to be effective, it is necessary for her to give birth to a live baby. Thirdly, the overall structure of her treatment requires her to receive strong anti-psychotic medication. The administration of that treatment has been necessarily interrupted by her pregnancy ... It is not, therefore, I think stretching language unduly to say that achievement of a successful outcome of her pregnancy is a necessary part of the overall treatment of her mental disorder.*

If there had been no need for restraint, it is arguable that the judge would have simply dealt with the matter on an 'incapacity to consent' basis, and would not have had recourse to section 63 of the 1983 Act.

In other cases the Mental Health Act 1983 has not been utilized by the court to justify treatment, with the pure 'best interests' test being preferred. That this is the better approach is common sense. In the Tameside case the patient was already detained under the Mental Health Act 1983, but in order to use section 63 in other cases it would first be necessary to detain the patient compulsorily.

The case of *re* MB [1997] concerned a patient with a needle phobia (as did that of *re* L (Patient: non-consensual treatment) [1997]) who was refusing to consent to anaesthesia before a Caesarean was performed. The court held that such a phobia resulted in her being (*per* Butler-Sloss LJ in *re* MB [1997]):

> ... *incapable of making a decision at all. She was at that moment suffering an impairment of her mental functioning which disabled her. She was temporarily incompetent.*

To prevent inconsistency in future cases concerning competence, the court set out a 10-point procedure to be adopted in future applications. This procedure from *re* MB [1997] has been incorporated into Department of Health Guidance (EL(97)32 dated 27 June 1997). Salient matters include:

> *(1) The court is unlikely to entertain an application for a declaration unless the capacity of the patient to consent to or refuse the medical intervention is at issue ...*
>
> *(3) Those in charge should identify a potential problem as early as possible so that both the hospital and patient can obtain legal advice.*
>
> *(4) It is highly desirable that, in any case where it is not an emergency, steps are taken to bring it before the court, before it becomes an emergency, to remove the extra pressure from the parties and the court and to enable proper instructions to be taken, particularly from the patient ...*
>
> *(8) There should in general be some evidence, preferably but not necessarily from a psychiatrist, as to the competence of the patient, if competence is in issue ...*
>
> *(10) In order to be in a position to assess a patient's best interests the judge should be provided, where possible and if time allows, with information about the circumstances of and relevant background material about the patient.*

All practitioners should be familiar with these guidelines, since they are essential for good medical and ethical practice.

The midwife's role and the relevance of birth plans

As this suggests, the role of the midwife is crucial in identifying any patients who may refuse treatment, necessitating application to a court. However, the midwife has a very important role in explaining treatment options to patients. The intervention of the midwife may overcome any refusal by the patient, or enable her to choose a more suitable treatment regime. The responsibilities and sphere of practice of the midwife, as set out in the *Midwives' Rules and Code of Practice* (UKCC, 1998), emphasize the need for midwives to discuss treatment options and in particular to explain any risk factors that may be present in the preferred treatment route.

Most women now agree a birth plan with the professionals, indicating the preferred birth method. However, this is not (in the majority of cases) stated to be guaranteed – it is more a 'wish list' than a perceived right, and in addition many birth plans do not highlight the treatment options that the patient does not want. However, it could be argued that treatment choices, or more correctly treatment refusals, within the birth plan should be taken as being binding on the medical team. This is so regardless of whether the patient is incompetent at the time the treatment needs to be administered.

Advance directives, or 'living wills' as they are known, are becoming more acceptable as a means to indicate treatment regimes that are acceptable or not to the maker of the 'will'. The legal validity of such documents is not really in dispute insofar as the 'will' purports to refuse certain treatment, or treatment in given situations. In *re* T (Adult: refusal of treatment) [1992], the principle was expressed thus (*per* Lord Donaldson):

> *If there is a distinction between a failure to consent and a refusal to consent, it is because a refusal can take the form of a declaration of intention never to consent in the future or never to consent in some future circumstances.*

This concept has been accepted and followed in later cases – for example, *re* C (Adult: refusal of treatment) [1994]. Any directive can only take effect when the maker loses the capacity to make treatment decisions, and the directive must be made whilst the patient is competent to make the decision. Certain aspects of treatment cannot be excluded – principally 'basic care'. It must be noted that currently there is some doubt regarding the exact meaning of 'basic care'. The British Medical Association, in its Code of Practice of April 1995 on Living Wills defined it as care required to keep the patient comfortable: medical treatment must only be undertaken if its sole or primary purpose is to assist the patient's comfort. By contrast, the Law Commission, in its consultation paper on Mental Incapacity (Law Comm No 231, 28 February 1995), defines basic care as being care 'to maintain bodily cleanliness and to alleviate severe pain and the provision of direct oral nutrition and hydration'.

In addition, there is a presumption that a living will is invalid if the maker is pregnant when the treatment is proposed or when the specified event occurs, unless the woman has expressly included the possibility of pregnancy within the statement.

For the midwife advising a woman on her treatment options, there are obvious consequences in relation to living wills. The midwife must clarify if the patient has already made such an advance directive, and explore the need to amend the statement to reflect the patient's new condition. If the patient does not have an existing advance directive, care needs to be taken when completing the birth plan. As Lord Donaldson points out, there is a distinction between a patient making no statement on a particular treatment, or failing to consent to it, and the patient clearly refusing to countenance the treatment. If a woman does object to certain treatments, for example an epidural, the midwife must explore whether the patient is refusing, or simply registering an objection. If the former, this has to be recorded and thereafter complied with, since it is legally binding; if the latter, an expression of desire, the statement would not be binding upon the healthcare team. In the wish to meet the requirements of the *Midwives' Rules and Code of Practice* (UKCC, 1998), and the duty to both mother and baby, it may be tempting to record all statements about treatment as 'expressions of desire'. If this is done, however, the midwife and any other medical practitioner may face litigation and the award of damages against them.

Children as pregnant patients

Returning to the beginning of this chapter, it will be recalled that those who are competent to consent to treatment are those individuals of full age and sound mind. Children, not being of full age, do not fall within the initial concept. Naturally the law has dealt with this – the basic principle is that where the patient is a minor (i.e. below 18 years of age), consent to treatment can be given by any person who has parental responsibility over the child. 'Parental responsibility' is a term introduced by the Children Act 1989, and refers to those persons who have rights, duties, powers, responsibility and authority over a child (s. 3(1)). In most cases this will be the biological parent, noting that an unmarried father does not automatically have these rights. Difficulties arise where a child is 'older' and able to make his or her own treatment decisions. For the midwife this is the norm, since most patients are over the age of 16 years. In this situation, the legal principle above has developed a gloss.

The starting point for the rights of the mature child to consent to treatment is the Family Law Reform Act 1969. Under s.8(1) of this Act:

> *The consent of a minor who has attained the age of sixteen years to any surgical, medical or dental treatment which, in the absence of consent, would constitute a trespass to his person, shall be as effective as it would be if he were of full age; and where a minor has by virtue of this section given an effective consent to any treatment it shall not be necessary to obtain any consent for it from his parent or guardian.*

Hence, once a child reaches the age of 16 years, he or she has a right to consent to treatment.

If the child is below 16 years of age, the 1969 Act is inapplicable. This is not to say that children below this age are never capable of consenting. In the well-publicized case of Gillick *v.* West Norfolk and Wisbech Area Health Authority [1986], the court held that a child could consent to treatment and that this was dependent upon:

> *... the minor having sufficient understanding and intelligence to make the decision and is not to be determined by reference to any judicially fixed age limit.*

In addition to the above, Lord Scarman stated that:

> *As a matter of law the parental right to determine whether or not their minor child below the age of 16 will have medical treatment terminates if and when the child achieves a sufficient understanding and intelligence to enable him or her to understand fully what is proposed.*

From this it would appear that the child, once in possession of the requisite degree of intelligence, gains individual autonomy. This autonomy presumably includes the right of the child to refuse treatment. However, the courts have subsequently limited this principle of autonomy. In the cases of *re* R (A minor: wardship: medical treatment) [1991] and *re* W (A minor: medical treatment) [1992], Lord Donaldson moved the law from a position of either the parent having the right to consent, or the child, to one of parallel rights. In Donaldson's view, when a child reached an age of sufficient understanding, whilst the child could consent, so could the parent (unless of course the Family Law Reform Act 1969 applied). On the issue of refusal of medical treatment, Donaldson held that whilst a child may refuse treatment, if a parent with a parallel right to consent agreed to that treatment, it could lawfully proceed. Where a child was over 16, the Family Law Reform Act 1969 did not provide total autonomy, since it only permitted the child to consent. The Act refers only to consent and not refusal. Therefore, under the interpretation of the law by Lord Donaldson, a child over 16 may refuse, but a parent still retains the right to consent, and treatment can then proceed lawfully.

A midwife with a child mother can therefore be seen to be in a difficult position with regard to treatment choices and options. If parent and child are in agreement, few problems are envisaged. Where they are not, the midwife needs to use all her skills to avoid conflict, but primarily this will be on a personal level. Insofar as the law is concerned, where the child patient is consenting to a form of treatment, if that is perceived to be acceptable, the midwife can proceed without fear of legal action if the child is judged competent. If the child is refusing but the parent is consenting, again the midwife can proceed, if treatment is perceived to be acceptable, without fear of legal action.

Implicit within this is the potential for a breach of the rules of confidentiality. If the duty is owed to the child patient, how will the parent find out what treatment has been discussed without the confidentiality being breached? Again, a midwife needs to exercise great care in these cases, and should make clear to the child patient that any information may have to be shared with the parents. It is always beneficial if the midwife can encourage the child to disclose voluntarily.

Reconciling conflicts with the *Midwives' Rules and Code of Practice*

The *Midwives' Rules and Code of Practice* (UKCC, 1998) has been mentioned at various points during the above discussion. The potential for conflict between the contents of these provisions where responsibilities and spheres of practice are concerned and the legal principles is one that any midwife in practice should be aware of. The midwife is, according to the code, responsible to the needs of the mother and baby. However, legally any responsibility must surely be to the mother alone since the fetus will have no rights until after birth. This proposition is somewhat ameliorated by the operation of the Congenital Disabilities (Civil Liabilities) Act 1976. Morally and ethically this may be contrary to the beliefs of many practising midwives. It is true to say that the relationship between ethics, morals and the law is one of tension, with the different bases for action pulling in opposite directions; if not diametrically opposed, they often do not pull together.

Conclusion

The ability to provide full and detailed information on all aspects of consent to treatment in such a short space is somewhat constrained. However, it is hoped that the discussion has at least highlighted some of the difficulties that exist when a woman is pregnant and receiving health care, primarily from her midwife. The key to avoiding many of the difficulties is the ability to establish a good working relationship between midwife and patient. That midwives are skilled in doing this is not in doubt, but there is always room for improvement where the giving of advice is concerned. Midwives should therefore pay careful attention to the wishes and desires of their patients, and bear in mind that the patient is nearly always right.

References

British Medical Association (1995). *Code of Practice on Living Wills.* BMA.
Law Commission (1995). *Mental Incapacity* (Law Comm No 231, 28 Feb).
The Telegraph (1993) **18 Jan**.
United Kingdom Central Council for Nursing, Midwifery and Health Visiting (1998). *Midwives' Rules and Code of Practice*. UKCC.

Legal cases:

Airedale NHS Trust *v.* Bland [1993] 1 All ER 821.
C *v.* S [1987] 1 All ER 1230.
Gillick *v.* West Norfolk and Wisbech Area Health Authority [1986] AC 112.
Mail Newspapers PLC *v.* Express Newspapers PLC [1987] Fleet Street Reports 91.
Norfolk and Norwich Healthcare (NHS) Trust *v.* W [1996] 2 F.L.R 613.
Paton *v.* Trustees of British Pregnancy Advisory Service [1978] 2 All ER 987.
Re C (Adult: refusal of treatment) [1994] 1 All ER 819.
Re F (In utero) [1988] 2 All ER 193.
Re F (Mental patient: sterilization) [1990] 2 A.C 1.
Re L (Patient: non-consensual treatment) *The Times* 1 January 1997.
Re MB [1997] 2 F.L.R 426.
Re R (A minor: wardship: medical treatment) [1991] 4 All ER 177.
Re S (Adult: refusal of medical treatment) [1993] 1 F.L.R 26.
Re T (Adult: refusal of treatment) [1992] 4 All ER 649.
Re W (A minor: medical treatment) [1992] 4 All ER 627.
Schloendorff *v.* Society of New York Hospital [1914] 211 NY 125.
Tameside and Glossop Acute Services Trust *v.* CH [1996] 1 F.L.R 762.

7

Genetic counselling: legal and ethical dilemmas

Jean McHale

Introduction

The advent of genetic screening has provided us with great potential. The knowledge of our genetic condition can enable us to avert illness. In a situation in which there is not a cure, it can enable an individual at least to plan for the future and make a particular decision. Screening may, however, equally give rise to considerable ethical dilemmas. Providing an individual with information regarding the prospects for the development of a late-onset condition may be as much burden as benefit (Advisory Committee on Genetic Testing, 1998). The very fact of screening may have future implications for insurance and employment prospects. A pregnant woman may find that the information gained as a result of genetic screening leads her to contemplate whether to have an abortion. This chapter explores the role of the law in this area in relation to the work of the midwife, focusing on the dilemmas and choices that may face the pregnant woman. First, the advantages and also some of the ethical dilemmas that may arise from the practice of genetic screening are considered. Secondly, some of the choices that may arise as a result of screening are explored. The prospect of liability in negligence consequent upon failure to undertake screening is considered; whether individuals who discover that they are at risk of giving birth to a child with genetic defects should refrain from reproducing is also discussed. Thirdly, the use that can be made of information uncovered as a result of genetic screening, and the dilemmas of disclosure that may ensue, are examined. The chapter focuses upon these issues in the context of the adult patient.

Genetic screening: the potential and the dilemmas

There are, broadly speaking, three categories of genetic disease:

1. Chromosomal disorders, which may arise either where an entire chromosome is added or missing, or where there has been rearrangement of chromosome material. Down's syndrome is an illustration of a chromosome disorder.
2. Unifactoral disease, such as cystic fibrosis and Huntington's chorea, which results from the presence of a specific abnormal gene. Where there is a family history it is possible to test selectively and to offer individuals advice and counselling. The genes may be autosomal dominants, which means that

they will express themselves as a pair of genes containing only one that is abnormal. Problems can arise should the onset of the disease occur later in life. If the gene is an autosomatic recessive, then the person with such a gene will carry it and disease will only result if both partners are carriers of the gene (e.g. cystic fibrosis). Some disorders are X-linked – i.e. sex-linked. Most occur only in males, who inherit the condition from their mothers. Unifactoral disease is frequently carried on one chromosome but not on another.

3. Multi-factoral (or polygenic) conditions, which arise as a result of both environmental factors and the presence of one or more of certain genes. For example, coronary heart disease appears to be genetically determined up to a certain point, but may also be influenced by a number of other factors. This relationship between gene and environmental factors is still largely unknown. Greater knowledge may enable healthcare professionals to target those individuals who may be at risk.

As the BMA has stated (BMA, 1992):

> *Genetic and pre-genetic diseases affect one in 20 by the age of 25 and perhaps as many as 2 in 3 people during their lifetime.*

The mapping of the human genome will have the effect that a complete 'book of life' for any particular individual can be compiled from a single cell biopsy. This will enable determination of whether an individual is a carrier, or has a slightly greater risk of developing a particular condition than applies to the population generally. Furthermore, susceptibilities to particular living conditions or environmental hazards will be revealed. As McLean (1995) comments:

> *... the more we find out about our genetic inheritance the more theoretically we can plan our lives, perhaps even avoid the illness which non-genetic factors might otherwise trigger.*

A woman may be included in a genetic screening programme prior to pregnancy, or she may decide to be screened or tested during pregnancy itself. While the terms 'screening' and 'testing' are at times used interchangeably, it is the case that diagnostic testing is the term used to describe the testing of an individual patient, while screening refers to procedures in which whole populations are tested on public health grounds or for research purposes. The Nuffield Council on Bioethics (para 1.10) defines genetic screening as:

> *... a search in a population to identify individuals who may have, or be susceptible to a serious genetic disease or who, though not at risk themselves as gene carriers may be at risk of having children with that genetic disease.*

Screening itself may take a number of forms. For example, an entire population may be screened where all groups within that population are at risk, or sub-groups within the population where the risk is known to be concentrated. Screening allows genetic disorders to be identified at an early age and thus may facilitate treatment. It may identify genetic susceptibility to particular common diseases, and may also assist in alleviating the anxieties of families and communities faced with the prospect of serious genetic disease. Screening enables couples to have a greater chance of making informed choices if they want to conceive children. Screening can be undertaken during pregnancy through the use of amniocentesis and chorion villus sampling, and screening of newborns may enable treatment of certain diseases. Screening may be undertaken with the aim of identifying whether a person currently has a disorder or whether he or she is a carrier or may, while not having the disease at present, in future develop the condition.

Despite the many perceived advantages that may accrue through screening, there are concerns regarding its practice. While testing can be a benefit, at times it can also be a burden. There is the risk of stigmatization where individuals are born with genetic conditions that have not been 'screened out'. The Nuffield Council on Bioethics stated that:

> It has been argued that the availability of prenatal screening and diagnosis together with the termination of seriously affected pregnancies both reflect and reinforce the negative attitudes of our society towards those with disabilities. Indeed medical genetics may add a new dimension if genetic disorder came to be seen as a matter of choice rather than fate.

The Nuffield Council on Bioethics was nonetheless of the view that at present this was unfounded fear. However, some commentators have subsequently highlighted the potential for discrimination. Society has indicated that discrimination against the disabled is unacceptable through the enactment of the Disability Discrimination Act 1995. However, genetic conditions are not included in the scope of the 1995 Act until the condition manifests itself.

Choices regarding screening

As with any other clinical procedure, it is necessary to obtain the consent of the patient before screening is undertaken. Failure to obtain consent will render the midwife liable in the tort of battery; the provision of inadequate information may give rise to liability in the law of negligence (see McHale *et al.*, 1998). An important element of consent is that it is both informed and voluntary (Science and Technology Committee, 1995a). The patient should not be directed into making the choice regarding genetic screening. The choices available that need to be explored and the consequent information provided relate to the point at which screening is proposed. The failure to provide information consequent upon genetic screening may lead to the healthcare professional being found liable in negligence (see Gregory *v.* Pembrokeshire [1989]).

If screening has been undertaken prior to conception, then the parties may consider use of new reproductive technologies to facilitate the screening out of genetic defects, or the use of sex selection. Some women who are unable to conceive naturally because of the prospect of passing on a genetic defect may still conceive through the use of artificial reproductive technologies. In 1998, the Human Fertilization and Embryology Authority ordered a report into the ethics of embryo screening for genetic defects (*The Times*, 1998; Human Fertilization and Embryology Authority, 1999). Pre-implantation genetic diagnosis enables the genetic condition to be screened out and avoids the prospect of a woman having to decide whether or not to have an abortion. Four centres are licensed at present under the Human Fertilization and Embryology Authority to undertake pre-implantation genetic diagnosis. Of these, only one centre is licensed for the purposes of performing an embryo biopsy. At present this is most commonly used in relation to the diagnosis of cystic fibrosis, and is also used in a situation where one partner is particularly at risk of transmitting a chromosome abnormality. However, the technique may be problematic. As the consultation paper issued by the Human Genetics Advisory Commission and the Human Fertilization and Embryology Authority noted, it may lead to loss of embryos owing to damage caused during biopsy, with the consequent impact that this may have upon a successful pregnancy. The use of pre-implantation genetic diagnosis is also linked to the success of *in vitro* fertilization (IVF) itself. The ethics of this technique are currently under debate. Some may regard it as ethically more acceptable in that disposal of an affected embryo is a matter of a different degree to disposal of a fetus in the later stages of pregnancy. Others, however, would disagree, arguing that the moral position of embryo and fetus cannot be so differentiated. The practical barriers to the use of pre-implantation genetic diagnosis – that is to say, its link with IVF – suggest that it is unlikely, at least for the considerable future, that such technology will become widespread.

The consultation document invited views as to what restrictions may be imposed upon those who may have access to pre-implantation genetic diagnosis. The document acknowledged that, in view of the developments in this area, the number of conditions for which pre-implantation genetic diagnosis was included should be subject to limitations. Consultation has been invited regarding whether the seriousness of the genetic condition should be a matter for clinical judgement, and also whether, at present, limitations should be imposed on the number and range of tests. A further issue is whether it would be correct deliberately to cause a child to be born with a disability, or whether, in the light of the knowledge that an embryo was infected, to continue with pregnancy. What if a woman, through screening, discovers that she is at risk of transmitting a genetic disorder and then continues with her pregnancy? Purdy (1996) has suggested that an individual may have a duty not to reproduce. She argues that persons with, for example, Huntington's chorea are unlikely to have what she terms 'minimally satisfying lives' and therefore those who may pass it on should not have genetically related children. She admits the difficulties in attempting to define a 'minimally satisfying life', but she goes on to say that there is no need to consider this complication at length here because we are concerned only with health as 'a prerequisite for a minimally satisfying life'. Alternatively, it can be argued that parents should try to secure something like normal health for their children. She states that such a position would still justify efforts to avoid the birth of children at risk for Huntington's disease and other serious genetic diseases in all societies. She admits that this may come into conflict with a 'right to reproduce', but suggests that there are other ways in which reproductive desires may be satisfied, including adoption and the use of new reproductive technologies. She comments that one of the arguments for having children, wanting the genetic line to be continued, is not particularly rational when it brings a sinister legacy of illness and death. The argument for having children on economic grounds – the cushion for old age – may not, she argues, provide the expected economic benefit if they are ill, and indeed 'expected economic benefit is, in many cases, a morally questionable reason for having children. She suggests that the 'right not to know' a genetic diagnosis can only be defended where this does not put others at risk.

However, others dispute this approach. A 'duty' not to reproduce may be seen as being in conflict with other recognized 'rights'. Elaine Sutherland suggested that to hold a woman liable for her decision to have a child despite substantial warnings regarding the risks of such a course of action might also constitute a breach of the European Convention on Human Rights – i.e. Article 12, the right to marry and found a family (Sutherland and McCall Smith, 1990). There are also fundamental questions regarding the privacy of the individual in relation to home and family life, under Article 8, which would arise in such a situation. The Council of Europe Convention on Bioethics provides, under Article 11, that 'Any form of discrimination against a person on grounds of his or her genetic heritage is prohibited'. We need, of course, to bear this in mind in relation to the Human Rights Act 1998. John Robertson, in his book *Children of Choice*, considers whether there is a case for compulsory contraception to prevent the birth of offspring with congenital disease or for persons who are HIV positive (this discussion is in connection with Norplant implants). He is of the view that both groups have substantial interests in reproduction. As he notes, in many situations the risk of bearing a handicapped child is only a fraction of that of giving birth to a healthy child in the same situation. In addition, some parents may be opposed to prenatal testing and abortion.

Certainly the imposition of a legal duty not to reproduce appears question-able, not least regarding the difficulties of judicial enforcement of such a duty. Use of the criminal law against those who decided to go ahead with pregnancy in the face of information that there was a high probability that the fetus would be born with some form of genetic disorder would be surely unthinkable. There would also be the prospect that the parents may be held accountable in civil law. At present, the potential for such actions is limited. While there is the possibility that fathers may be sued under the Congenital Disabilities Civil Liability Act 1976, mothers are excluded from liability with the exception of the situation where the mother has been involved in a road traffic accident (Brazier, 1997). While in 1976 limiting actions under the Act could be seen in terms of quite restricted notions of paternal misconduct, such as a man assaulting his pregnant partner, today medical science makes everything so much more complex. In practice, as Brazier says, to establish liability at present it is necessary to show that there is a duty to the mother, but in many of these instances outlined above, at the stage at which that happens the mother and child will have never met.

A child who is born with a genetic disorder may seek to argue in the courts that this birth was wrongful and that there should be liability in criminal law. Should a child be able to bring a 'wrongful life' action at all? Such an action was rejected in McKay v. Essex AHA [1982]. Mary McKay was born in 1975. She had been infected in the womb with rubella (German measles), and as a result she was partially blind and deaf. The allegation was made by the child that one doctor had acted negligently in failing to treat rubella infection on being told it was suspected. It was also claimed that another doctor had either negligently mislaid the blood sample or had failed to interpret the results of blood tests. The real issue in the case was that the doctor owed the plaintiff a duty of care when she was *in utero*, which involved advising her mother as to the desirability of having an abortion – advice the mother said she would have accepted. The Court of Appeal rejected her claim. Acker LJ said that there was a whole series of undesirable consequences that would result from a wrongful birth claim being allowed. First, if the duty of care to the fetus involved imposing a duty on the doctor – albeit indirectly – to prevent the child's birth, the child would have a cause of action against the mother if she refused to have an abortion. Second, how could a court attempt to evaluate non-existence? The undiscovered country from whose lands no traveller returns would make it difficult to try to compare non-existence (the doctor alleged to be negligent having deprived her of this) and the value of her existence in a disabled state. Stephenson LJ said that the claim was in effect that there was a duty to abort the unborn child. The fact that a doctor can lawfully terminate life didn't mean that the child had a right to die, and to recognize such a right would be contrary to public policy. The only duty of care that could be recognized in this case was one that could be assessed in monetary terms; how can courts assess the difference between conduct as a result of their allowing the fetus to be born alive although injured, as compared with its condition if its embryonic life had been ended before its life in the world had begun? He noted the rejection of the wrongful life claim the in USA in the case of Gleitman *v.* Cosgrave [1967], where the court had said that in assessing damages the problem was that of question of whether X would have been better off not being born at all:

> Man who knows nothing of death or nothingness cannot possibly know whether that is so.

The Law Commission, in its *Report on Injuries to Unborn Children*, rejected the wrongful life claim. It was of the view that it would impose an intolerable burden on the medical profession because of subconscious pressure to advise abortion in doubtful cases because of the fear of action for damages. Interestingly, Griffith LJ did not see this as a tenable ground. He was of the view that provided the defendants gave a balanced explanation of risks involved in alleged pregnancy, including risk of injury to the fetus, the doctor couldn't be expected to do more. He saw the most insoluble problem as the assessment of damages. The court had to compare the plaintiff's state with a non-existence, regarding which the court can know nothing. He also said that section 1(5) of the Congenital Disabilities (Civil Liability) Act 1976 excluded liability in wrongful life claims – a point on which all the members of the Court of Appeal in this case agreed. Section 4(5) of the 1975 Act provides that the Act applies to all births after its passing and in respect of any such birth it replaces any law in force before its passage whereby a person could be held liable to a child in respect of disabilities with which it might be born.

The difficulties that arise in the context of the competent adult are magnified still further when considering mentally incompetent persons or teenage pregnancy. Should teenagers be penalized whether or not they know of the risk they may be under with regard to conception? What about the overlap with abortion once a woman discovers that she is carrying a handicapped infant during pregnancy? As Brazier (1997) has commented:

> A woman who appreciating the risk that her child would suffer from that congenital disorder refused screening, or refused an abortion after a positive test, would be perceived by some commentators as having culpably caused a child to be born disabled. Her maternal conduct would be perceived as analogous to the woman who did nothing to diminish her abuse of addictive drugs.

At present, the consequences of such a duty not to reproduce are such that it is unlikely that the courts would be willing to impose such a duty upon the parents.

Some concerns have arisen regarding the use of sex-selection techniques that may be used as a consequence of genetic screening. The Council of Europe Convention on Bioethics and Human Dignity provides, in Article 14, that:

> The use of techniques of medically assisted procreation shall not be allowed for the purpose of choosing a future child's sex, except where serious hereditary sex-related disease is to be avoided.

If screening is undertaken and there is a high probability or some risk that a child will be born with a genetic condition that may develop in the future, the pregnant woman may seek an abortion. The Abortion Act 1967 sanctions an abortion where two medical practitioners are satisfied that one of the grounds for abortion under the Act has been complied with. The woman seeking an abortion following genetic screening is perhaps most likely to seek an abortion under sections 1(1)a or 1(1)(d). Section 1(1)(a) is the subsection that sanctions so-called 'social abortions'. Here, abortion may be undertaken if the continuance of the pregnancy would involve greater risk to her physical or mental health, or to any existing children, than if the pregnancy were terminated. The time limit is currently fixed at 24 weeks, but the statute does not state when this period actually commences, and the legal position is unclear. It is also uncertain to what extent this subsection would, for example, encompass a decision to terminate on the basis of the sex of the fetus. Section 1(1)(d) allows abortion up until birth on the grounds of fetal handicap. It is unclear what severity of handicap gives rise to a right to an abortion under this section (Morgan, 1990), and whether it includes those handicaps that a child will be born with if the pregnancy continues, or whether it also covers those genetic conditions (such as Huntington's chorea) where the onset of the condition is not until the third or fourth decade of life.

In many situations genetic diagnosis by itself will not be conclusive regarding whether an individual will develop or pass on a particular disorder (Mason and McCall Smith, 1999):

> ... the counsellor can virtually never make a firm statement as to having or not having a further child. He can take extraneous circumstances – e.g. religious or financial status – into consideration, but, in the end, he is down to speaking about probabilities. In the case of unifactoral disease he can give accurate figures – i.e. if both the mother and the father carry recessive deleterious genes, the chance of an overtly affected child is one in four pregnancies.

As technology is advancing, there may be the possibility of a cure for some genetic diseases in the future. The parents, in making their decision, must be adequately counselled as to the alternatives.

Confidentiality of information gained in screening

Further dilemmas may arise regarding the confidentiality of information obtained through genetic screening. For instance, the healthcare professional justified in disclosing information gained during genetic screening to third parties? For example, take the woman who is screened during pregnancy. This information may be of assistance to her sister, who is also contemplating pregnancy. The woman may of course be perfectly happy for the information to be disclosed to her sister, with the suggestion being made to the sister that she should also be screened. However, she may not. In such a situation, could the midwife legitimately take the decision to breach the patient's confidentiality?

The midwife is subject to an obligation of confidentiality, both in law and under the midwives' professional ethical code. The UKCC requires that the practitioner must

> ... *protect all confidential information of patients and clients obtained in the course of professional practice and make disclosures only with consent, where required by the order of the court or where you can justify disclosure in the general public interest.*

Should the midwife breach confidentiality without authority, he or she may be subject to professional disciplinary procedures. English law also requires that confidentiality of healthcare information should be protected, primarily through the operation of the equitable remedy of breach of confidence. The Law Commission (1981) has described this as being:

> ... *a civil remedy affording protection against disclosure or use of information which is not publicly known and which has been entrusted to a person in circumstances importing an obligation not to disclose or use that information without the authority of the person who imparted it.*

The courts have confirmed that such an obligation arises by virtue of the healthcare professional–patient relationship. In X v. Y [1988], talking in the context of HIV, Rose J stated that:

> *In the long run preservation of confidentiality is the only way of securing public health: otherwise doctors would not be discredited as a source of education, for future patients will not come forward if doctors are going to squeal on them.*

The obligation of confidence is not absolute; the public interest in maintaining confidentiality may be outweighed by the public interest in disclosure (see Attorney General v. Guardian Newspapers [1988]). In determining whether or not certain disclosures are in the public interest, the courts have indicated that they are prepared to take note of guidance issued by the profession on this matter (UKCC, 1996):

> *The public interest means the interests of an individual, or groups of individuals or society as a whole, would, for example, cover matters such as serious crime, child abuse, drug trafficking or other activities which place others at serious risk.*

As will be seen below, it may be very difficult indeed to establish the basis on which disclosure of genetic information may be justified in the public interest.

The issue of public interest

When can and should the right to keep genetic information secret be outweighed by the public interest in disclosure? While relatives have no right to discover details regarding a person's medical history, in some situations the disclosure of genetic information may be justifiable – for example, if the relative is at risk of developing a particular condition and it is possible that this condition could be prevented through potential environmental factors or by late in life, and, if they had known about it, was a risk that they could have avoided.

The question remains as to how the courts will interpret the boundaries of public interest in such a situation. In the past, cases have focused on matters such as whether harm will be caused. But can harm here be easily detected? It could be that disclosure of information may lead to someone else being tested, and a treatable condition thereby diagnosed. At present this is subject to a limited number of categories. It should not be forgotten that as far as most genetic disorders are concerned, an important factor is not whether such risks *will* develop but the fact that such a risk *could* develop. However, the situation may not be that clear-cut. It may be the case simply that there is a risk that the person screened will develop a particular condition.

Should a pregnant woman be given information gained through the genetic screening of a relative? In this situation, can disclosure ever be justified on the basis that it is to avoid harm being caused to others, the disclosure being in the public interest? In the case of the pregnant woman, it has indeed been suggested that the matter is really whether there is a loss of opportunity to benefit. As Boddington (1994) has commented, this differs substantially from those situations where the disclosure relates to infectious disease. The emphasis is not on harm to the individual as such, but may mean that the population is protected from bearing the costs of persons with genetic conditions. Unlike many diseases, the issue of genetic disease cannot be regarded in terms of the same manner of diseases being transmitted within the population as a whole.

In considering disclosure, the Nuffield Council on Bioethics suggests that two factors are relevant – the consequence of the refusal to supply the information, and the reason why an individual refuses permission. It may be the case that the reason for refusal of disclosure is malicious, but at the same time it could be the case that disclosure would reveal compromising information about paternity. Finally, there is a risk that disclosure could harm the woman not only because of the breach of confidentiality but also because of the impact on the relationship with the man involved.

Should persons have a legal duty to disclose their own genetic information to others?

To what extent should patients have a responsibility to make a voluntary disclosure of their own genetic information? The Nuffield Council on Bioethics comments that a person acting responsibly would normally communicate such information, and indeed it can be said that it is the primary obligation of that person so to do. The Council rejected a legally enforceable duty, and indicated that in any event considerable difficulties might arise in relation to attempts to enforce any such duty – how, for example, could family members enforce it? Moreover (Nuffield Council on Bioethics, para 5.27):

> *In any event in certain circumstances there may be perfectly good reasons why an individual would not wish to inform family members about the result of a genetic test. For example, a woman who has discovered that she is a carrier for Duchenne muscular dystrophy may not wish at that time to tell her sister who is seven months' pregnant.*

As noted, while sharing information with family members may be regarded as the best approach, the Nuffield Council on Bioethics states that disclosure within the family unit ought not to be a condition of participation in screening (para 5.26). Usually people will be willing to share this information amongst their family and extended family, but if they are not willing, can the healthcare professional break confidence and disclose? In the case of genetic screening, it may be that the boundaries of disclosure of such information have been agreed in advance before the process of screening itself is undertaken. This form of 'negotiated confidentiality' is akin to the model adopted in social work, and has received a modicum of support from certain sections of the medical profession (Thompson, 1979). However, the use of such negotiation has been questioned by some commentators, who suggest that it may be undesirable, and indeed regarded as coercion, to make such agreement a condition of the screening itself being undertaken.

In such situations, is it a desirable approach to look beyond the principle of individual confidentiality and consider the context of the whole family? If genetic information is seen in terms of being in some form of common owner-ship, then this would limit any individual's right to control the passage of that information. The Nuffield Council on Bioethics noted that in certain clearly defined contexts it might be appropriate to treat the family as a unit. It suggested that where disease would cause grave danger to family members, an attempt should be made to ensure that the information was disclosed voluntarily. In exceptional situations information could be disclosed by healthcare profes-sionals to other family members despite an expressed wish for confidentiality, if for example it was to avoid giving rise to grave damage to family members. The recommendation of the Council of Europe follows the same lines:

> *Communication of unexpected findings to family members of the person tested should only be authorized by national law if the person tested refuses expressly to release information although the life of the family member may be in danger.*

Genetic registers are defined by the Nuffield Council on Bioethics as being a collection of relevant information on individuals who have particular genetic diseases, and may also include information regarding relatives who may be at risk of developing the condition. They may operate as a starting point for genetic screening. Alternatively, a register may act as a basis for screening when that register is not specifically genetic in its nature. A genetic register may be the result of a genetic screening programme. As the Nuffield Council on Bioethics (para 5.35) quite rightly notes, it is of importance for individuals to be aware that their information is contained in such a register. The Council recommended that:

> *... in such circumstances health professionals should seek to persuade individuals if persuasion should be necessary to allow the disclosure of relevant genetic information to other family members.*

As far as healthcare professionals are concerned, would the law impose upon them any liability for non-disclosure to third parties of information discovered through screening? This would appear unlikely, although in the USA courts have imposed liability upon healthcare professionals for failure to disclose informa-tion to third parties that may have enabled them to avert harm. The imposition of such a duty in English law is unlikely. As has been suggested, such a duty would not only place the healthcare professional in the position of having to work out whether or not to break confidentiality, but would also result in the difficult situation of deciding whether in effect he or she is infringing the third party's right not to know (HermanNys).

While the Science and Technology Committee has noted that there are some examples of cases in which children have been born with a handicap who would not otherwise have been born had relatives shared their genetic knowledge, nevertheless it is of the view that confidence should not be broken, stating that:

> *If genetic tests are desirable for individual or public health reasons people should be able to take them without the fear that their genetic constitution will be revealed to others.*

(Science and Technology Committee, 1995, para 227)

Nevertheless, the Committee does recommend that, wherever possible, counsellors should try to convince those persons who are being tested as to the desirability of administering the tests. They suggest that relatives could be approached through the GP being given names and addresses of those tested, and the GP then approaching the relatives. However, this may be difficult in practice. There is also one further consideration, which is that third parties may not actually want to know their genetic diagnosis. It has been suggested that there may be a right not to know such information, to remain in ignorance of it (Chadwick *et al*, 1998). The Convention for the Protection of Human Rights and Dignity of the Human Being with regard to the application of Biology and Medicine, Article 10(2), states that:

> *Everyone is entitled to know any information collected about his or her health. However the wishes of individuals not so to be informed should be observed.*

Observing these countervailing 'rights' may give rise to some very difficult questions of clinical judgement.

Conclusions

Genetic counselling can facilitate choices consequent upon pregnancy, but these choices bring with them responsibilities for healthcare professionals. Fundamental questions of public policy also arise in such situations. This chapter has given an overview of some of the choices and dilemmas that may arise in relation to the work of the midwife. The House of Commons Select Committee on Science and Technology recommended that a Human Genetics Commission should be established. The Human Genetics Advisory Commission, which was established in 1996, is concerned with issues of genetics that lie primarily outside health care. Its scope has covered, for example, the relationship of genetics and employment and insurance matters. The Advisory Committee on Genetic Testing has been operational since 1995 (Science and Technology Committee, 1995b). It is a non-statutory body, and its terms of reference are to provide advice to ministers on developments in testing for genetic disorders; to advise on testing individuals for genetic disorders taking account of ethical, social and scientific aspects; and to establish requirements, especially in terms of efficacy and product information, to be met by manufacturers and suppliers of genetic tests. In December 1998, the government announced its intention to review the regulation of biotechnological developments. The decision was made to establish a Human Genetics Commission (HGC) to undertake strategic analysis, and to provide advice and guidance to ministers in the light of international and European developments. It will take over the work of existing bodies, such as the Human Genetics Advisory Commission. However, while some guidance can be given, it is necessarily the case that we are looking at a moving target in the light of constantly changing scientific developments. Moreover, the legal regulation of this area is likely to be only in the most general terms. Midwives and other healthcare professionals will need to monitor legal and regulatory developments closely, and reassess their position accordingly on a regular basis.

References

Advisory Committee on Genetic Testing (1998). *Report on Genetic Testing for Late Onset Disorders.*

Boddington, P. (1994). Confidentiality and genetic counselling. In: *Genetic Counselling: Principles and Practice* (A. Clarke, ed.), p. 236. Routledge.

Brazier, M. (1997). Parental responsibilities, fetal welfare and children's health. In: *Family Law, Towards the Millennium* (C. Bridge, ed.). Butterworths.

British Medical Association (1992). Oxford University Press.

Chadwick, R., Levitt, M. and Shickle, D. (1998). *The Right to Know and the Right Not to Know.* Avebury.

Cunningham, J., Meacher, M., Jowell, T. *et al.* (1999). T*he Advisory and Regulatory Framework for Biotechnology: Report from the Government's Review*, p. 17. Cabinet Office, Office of Science and Technology.

Human Fertilization and Embryology Authority and Advisory Committee on Genetic Testing (1999). Consultation Document on Pre-implantation Genetic Diagnosis.

Law Commission (1974). *Report on Injuries to Unborn Children*, No 60.

Law Commission (1981). *Breach of Confidence.* Cmnd 8388, p. 10.

Mason, J. K. and McCall Smith, R. A. (1999). *Law and Medical Ethics*, 5th edn. Butterworth's

McHale, J., Tingle, J. and Peysner, J. (1998). *Law and Nursing*, Chapters 5 and 6. Butterworth-Heinemann.

McLean, S. (1995). *Science's Holy Grail – Some Legal and Ethical Implications of the Human Genome Project.* CLP 232.

Morgan, D. (1990). Abortion: the unexamined ground? *Criminal Law Rev.*, 687.

Nuffield Council on Bioethics, www.nuffieldfoundation.org.bioethics.

Purdy, L. (1996) *Reproducing Persons Issues in Feminist Bioethics*, pp. 43–48. Cornell University Press.

Robertson, J. (1994). *Children of Choice*, Princeton University Press.

Science and Technology Committee (1995a). The BMA's view on genetic testing. House of Lords Select Committee on Science and Technology Committee, 3rd Report; para 81–105.

Science and Technology Committee (1995b). *Human Genetics: the Science and Its Consequence.*

Sutherland, E. and McCall Smith, R. A. (1990). Regulating pregnancy: should we and can we? In: *Family Rights and Family Responsibilities* (E. Sutherland and R. A. McCall Smith, eds). Edinburgh University Press.

The Times (1998). Designer baby inquiry ordered. **17 Jan**.

Thompson (1979). The nature of confidentiality. *J. Med. Ethics*, 5.

United Kingdom Central Council for Nurses, Midwives and Health Visitors (1996). *Guidelines for Professional Practice.* UKCC.

Legal cases:

Attorney General *v.* Guardian Newspapers (No 2) [1988] 3 All ER 545.
Gleitman *v.* Cosgrave 296 NYS 2d 687 [1967].
Gregory *v.* Pembrokeshire [1989] 1 Med LR 81.
McKay *v.* Essex AHA [1982] 2 All ER 771.
X *v.* Y [1988] 3 All ER 545.

8

The tools of risk management and their application to midwifery practice

Josie Williams

Introduction

Risk management is a systematic process, the principles of which should be incorporated into the practice of each midwife. This process is continuous, and is also a quality issue, with the reduction of risk resulting in the provision of higher quality midwifery care.

Ideally, risk management is undertaken in a proactive way so that action can be taken to prevent any injury or loss occurring. A reactive approach can be taken also to minimize the adverse outcomes of clinical incidents and to prevent, where possible, their recurrence. The tools discussed in this chapter are applicable to both types of risk management.

The risk management process should (NHSME, 1993):

- Address the various activities of an organization
- Identify the risks that exist
- Assess those risks for potential frequency and severity

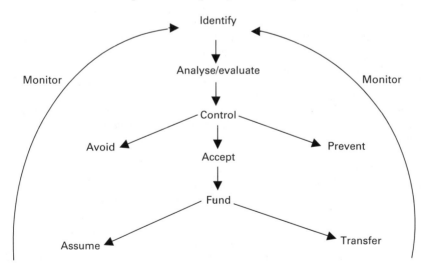

Figure 8.1 The risk management process (courtesy of D. Bowden, personal communication).

- Eliminate the risks that can be eliminated
- Reduce the effect of risks that cannot be eliminated
- Put into place financial mechanisms to absorb the financial consequences of the risks that remain.

Risk management can be broken down into three key stages:

1. Risk identification
2. Risk analysis
3. Risk control.

Although for the purposes of this chapter the various tools used in each stage are considered separately, it must be emphasized that this remains a continuous process which, like the audit cycle, is subject to ongoing monitoring and review (Figure 8.1).

Risk identification

Risk identification is the key to successful risk management. The aim is to determine:

- What could go wrong
- How it could happen
- What outcomes could result.

The concept of risk assessment is an essential part of midwifery practice, where it is important to identify any risks present in the care of a particular woman and her baby (Alexander and Keirse, 1989). However, whilst this concentrates on the individual, in risk management the identification process examines the physical environment, working practices and the organization in its entirety. This assessment concentrates on the systems in place to minimize risk, as well as identifying the risk factors involved in any clinical incidents or near misses reported.

The assessment should be undertaken in a systematic way, and may be performed by the Trust risk manager, appropriately trained and experienced midwives, or external consultants. An initial survey covering all the above areas will provide a baseline 'snapshot' of the risks present, thus facilitating the drafting of an action plan to address them. Subsequent assessments may be delegated to line managers or other specific individuals once they have received the necessary education and training to enable them to undertake this.

Preparation

Before any risk identification assessments are undertaken, the assessor needs to determine the criteria against which the degree of risk present can be assessed. Maternity care has a comprehensive set of nationally recognized standards that can be used as benchmarks for this purpose. These include the *Minimum Standards for the Organisation of Labour Wards* agreed by a joint working party of the Royal College of Midwives and the Royal College of Obstetricians and Gynaecologists (RCOG and RCM, 1999). In England, there are the *Clinical Risk Management Standards* of the Clinical Negligence Scheme for Trusts (CNST,

1999), which contain both general risk management standards and, in Standard 12, criteria specific to maternity care. The Welsh Risk Pool (1999) has *Risk Management Standards* that also refer to both general risk management standards and speciality-specific criteria (in Standard 12A). A similar risk pool (the Clinical Negligence and Other Risks Indemnity Scheme – CNORIS) has been commenced in Scotland.

In addition to the above criteria, the assessor may include unit-specific clinical indicators highlighted through the incident reporting system, complaints, or, indeed, claims against the Trust (see below).

There are a number of risk management tools available. Although each of these can be used in isolation, it is normal practice to utilize the more effective tools in conjunction with each other on an ongoing basis.

Questionnaires

Questionnaires can be used either as a stand-alone tool, or as part of a broader risk management survey. The content can be designed to determine whether systems are in place to meet the criteria in the previously agreed risk management standards; to ascertain the extent of compliance with these systems; and to assess staff perception of risk.

The main advantage of questionnaires is anonymity, which may persuade staff to give more honest answers than they may feel able to do in the perceived vulnerability of a face-to-face interview. It is also possible to include a far greater number of individuals in the risk assessment process, with the use of a structured questionnaire theoretically making the findings more valid statistically.

However, great care needs to be taken in the compilation of a questionnaire to ensure that the meaning of each question is unambiguous and not open to misinterpretation. This can be a time-consuming process, as is the analysis of those documents returned. The main disadvantage is the likelihood of a low response rate. This may affect the validity of the exercise, particularly if the respondents are not a truly representative sample of the staff group surveyed.

If there is sufficient time and funding available to undertake a questionnaire survey, this should be organized to take place at the beginning of the risk assessment process. This provides useful background data that can be used to inform subsequent parts of the assessment. It raises awareness amongst staff, which is helpful if they are required to participate in other aspects of the exercise, and may also stimulate their interest in the principles of risk management.

An initial questionnaire survey can also be used as a benchmark against which to measure the progress of the unit with regard to the particular questions being asked. This can be demonstrated by repeating the survey, using the same questionnaire, after a specified period and/or at regular intervals.

Checklists

These can be used to determine if particular risk factors are present, to verify whether specific control measures are in place, and to ascertain the degree of compliance with them. Provided that both their content and findings are validated by a suitably experienced and competent person, the completion of a checklist can be delegated to more junior staff. However, this approach, and indeed the use of checklists in general, can result in risk factors not included on the list being overlooked. Therefore they are utilized best in conjunction with other risk management tools rather than in isolation.

Documentation review

A comprehensive and ongoing review of policies, procedures, protocols and guidelines, together with regular audit of record-keeping standards, is an essential part of risk management. This topic is covered in depth in Chapter 2.

Observation and physical inspection

The assessor can identify a number of risks by walking round and inspecting a clinical area and informally talking with staff. It is preferable that inspection be undertaken by an individual who does not routinely work in that area, as familiarity with the environment may cause some risks to be overlooked.

Whilst the initial inspection may be organized centrally (e.g. by the Trust risk manager), subsequent inspections, which should be undertaken not less frequently than annually, may be delegated through the line management structure to appropriately trained midwives. This is commonly one of the responsibilities of the ward/team manager, with support provided by the risk manager. In order to overcome the challenge of over-familiarity with the area, it has been found helpful for managers to work in pairs, each inspecting the other's area of responsibility.

It can be beneficial if the person conducting the inspection is accompanied by a relatively new team member from the area being inspected. Not only does this provide someone to answer any queries, it also gives the assessor an insight into the working practices and communication within that clinical area. This can be very revealing, with information often gleaned that would not emerge in a more formalized interview situation. It is also educational for the team member involved.

Interviews

Face-to-face interviews, although time consuming, are a valuable source of information for the risk assessor. Areas covered should include working practices; knowledge of the various risk management systems in place; and adherence to agreed policies, procedures, protocols and guidelines. It is essential to gain the confidence of the interviewee, who must in turn feel able to trust that the interviewer will respect that confidence and not reveal the source of the information obtained. For that reason the interview should not be conducted by, or in the presence of, the interviewee's line manager. At the same time the interviewee, particularly if a junior member of staff, needs to feel empowered to talk to the interviewer about confidential matters. This is especially relevant if external consultants are used. This can be addressed by using staff meetings to give general information about the process in advance, with those selected for interview also being sent letters individually inviting their co-operation and giving information regarding the format and likely content of the interview.

A representative cross-section of staff should be selected. In order to gain maximum benefit, as well as reducing demands on the time of busy staff, a semi-structured format makes best use of the time allocated. Preparation is crucial to ensure that all relevant topics are covered. Time must be allowed also during which interviewees can raise perceived risk factors of particular concern to themselves. It is often at the end of the interview, when the interviewee is relaxing, that crucial information is volunteered.

It is important that related interviews cover the same topics, so that the information given can be cross-checked and verified. If possible, documentary evidence should be obtained to support the statements made. It is not unknown for interviewees to attempt to use the process to further their own personal agenda.

Grids

One of the simplest systems of identifying risks is to draft a grid matrix of hazards and targets (Figure 8.2). This is a 'paper exercise' that can be under-taken by a group of midwives, and is a useful method of raising awareness of risk. This is easier to use with regard to non-clinical risks, but could be adapted for any type of risk.

Flow charts

Flow charts are used to show in a systematic way the various stages or 'flow' in a process involving people, services, goods and materials (Figure 8.3). This demonstrates the inputs and outputs of the different stages, and identifies the dependencies and bottlenecks that pose a potential risk to the process as a

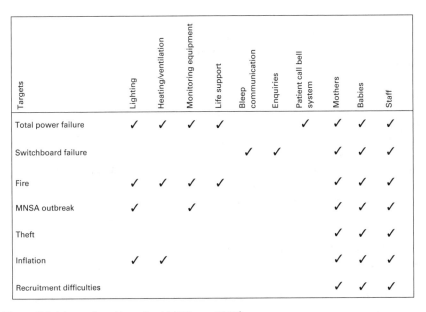

Targets	Lighting	Heating/ventilation	Monitoring equipment	Life support	Bleep communication	Enquiries	Patient call bell system	Mothers	Babies	Staff
Total power failure	✓	✓	✓	✓			✓	✓	✓	✓
Switchboard failure					✓	✓		✓	✓	✓
Fire	✓	✓	✓	✓				✓	✓	✓
MNSA outbreak	✓		✓					✓	✓	✓
Theft								✓	✓	✓
Inflation	✓	✓						✓	✓	✓
Recruitment difficulties								✓	✓	✓

Figure 8.2 A hazard and target grid (Wilson, 1999).

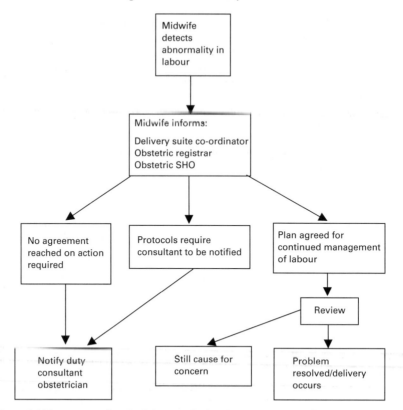

Figure 8.3 The process for obtaining medical assistance in labour (hospital delivery).

whole. Although of some use in midwifery, in many instances an alternative would be the implementation of multidisciplinary pathways of care (see Chapter 2).

Hazard and operability study

Hazard and operability studies (HAZOPs) are used particularly in the chemical industry, where processes are so complex that analysis is only feasible for component parts, which may in themselves be multifaceted. Although of possible use in the pathology laboratories, HAZOPs are not really appropriate to midwifery, and the method is included here only for the sake of completeness.

The technique involves:

- Describing the intention of a specified part of the process (e.g. flow or temperature)
- Identifying possible deviations from that intention (e.g. more/less)
- Listing all possible causes of each such deviation
- Evaluating the consequences of each cause
- Specifying the action necessary to control these consequences.

This produces a qualitative result, and is a useful aid in developing checklists for later use by others. Perhaps most importantly, it points towards the areas where the impact of a specific event would be greatest. However, a HAZOP study requires the involvement of a team of technical experts over an extended period of time, and is consequently costly.

Clinical incident reporting

Adverse events have been defined as 'incidents in which a patient is unintentionally harmed by {medical} treatment' (Vincent *et al.*, 1998). The reporting of such events, or 'clinical incidents' as they are increasingly called, underpins the whole process of clinical risk management. There are four essential aspects to this process:

- Acceptance of the need for reporting
- Knowing what to report
- Knowing how to report
- A system for collecting and collating the incidents reported.

Two types of incident are reported: poor outcomes, in which actual harm resulted; and 'near misses', where something untoward occurred but the outcome was unaffected on that occasion.

The management of poor outcomes was introduced originally as part of the claims management process, but is now seen also as having 'the potential to act as a gateway into a problem of much greater importance, that of injury to patients, which current quality initiatives have not adequately addressed' (Vincent, 1997). It is also being recognized that considerable support needs to be given to women, their families and the staff involved in such incidents (Genn, 1995; Vincent, 1995). The use of a debriefing system to help women understand what occurred during their labour and to question its management has been shown to help in this respect (Smith and Mitchell, 1996). The development of reflective thinking (Miller, 1999), together with support from colleagues and management, can benefit the midwives involved in any such occurrence.

It is essential that all clinical incidents are reported and investigated fully, both to manage any harm suffered and to allow action to be taken to prevent any future recurrence. For this to be successful, staff must feel empowered to report freely and without fear of disciplinary action being taken against them. The importance of this has been recognized by the CNST (1999; Criterion 4.1.9) and the Welsh Risk Pool (1999; Standard 3(v)).

Early reporting of clinical incidents allows the following action to be taken:

- Management of the incident
- Correction of any errors
- Minimization of any danger or distress
- Management of any consequent claim for damages
- Reduction in the risk of recurrence.

The inclusion of 'near misses' in the clinical incident reporting system demonstrates clearly that proactive risk management in particular is a quality issue. Based on the premise that 'improving quality in health care should include removing the causes of harm' (Vincent, 1997), reporting instances of failure to meet specific standards (e.g. decision to incision time for emergency Caesarean sections) allows action to be taken to address any underlying deficiencies in the system before any harm has resulted.

Hospitals and Trusts invariably have a centralized system for reporting clinical incidents Indeed, this is one of the key standards of both the CNST (1999; Standard 4) and the Welsh Risk Pool (1999; Standard 3). This system should include the reporting of near misses. Maternity units are often in the forefront of these developments, with, in most cases, the unit developing its own clinical indicators for reporting through the centralized system. However, some units have implemented their own system for reporting clinical incidents as part of a maternity unit clinical risk management process (Dineen, 1996; O'Connor and Beard, 1996).

The clinical indicators used should be agreed by both medical and midwifery staff. These may be derived from data obtained from investigation of previous claims against the Trust; from risks highlighted through the incident reporting system; from the results of clinical audit projects; and from standards set by the National Institute for Clinical Excellence (NICE) or other comparable standards. Whilst there is some variation between Trusts as to the indicators used, those listed in Tables 8.1 and 8.2 would usually be included.

The actual criteria to be used are often the subject of some debate amongst

Table 8.1 Clinical indicators for reporting: maternal

- Maternal death
- Admission to ITU
- Eclampsia
- Ruptured uterus
- Third-degree tear or damage to bladder
- Post-partum haemorrhage of < 1 litre
- Anaesthetic problem
- Failed forceps/ventouse delivery
- Prolonged second stage of over 3 hours
- Decision to incision interval of over 30 minutes for an emergency Caesarean section
- Unplanned return to the operating theatre
- Unattended delivery
- Refusal of treatment and/or complaint from client or family
- Delay in obtaining medical assistance

Table 8.2 Clinical indicators for reporting: fetal/neonatal

- Intrapartum stillbirth
- Unexpected admission to the neonatal unit
- Apgar score of < 7 at 5 minutes
- Birth injury
- Difficulty or delay in resuscitation
- Neonatal death
- Re-admission to the neonatal unit or to hospital
- Transfer to another unit/hospital

the clinicians leading the risk management process. Persuading staff to complete 'yet more forms' is one of the challenges of risk management, and an education programme for staff is an essential prerequisite to their introduction. It has been suggested (Capstick, 1994) that in order to achieve compliance with the system, the number of reportable indicators should be kept to a minimum. Whilst this remains an important consideration, experience of the systems in use in a number of maternity units suggests that staff tend to report only the indicators listed in the reporting protocol. Consequently, short lists tend to grow.

Incidents are usually reported on specially designed forms. Although traditionally paper-based, in Trusts with a comprehensive intranet a computerized system can be installed. This allows staff to enter information directly onto the system from a ward/department-based terminal. As well as making the information available immediately to the risk manager, such a system can link the clinical incident reports to the complaints management system, data from both of which being available to the claims manager. This allows a proactive approach to be taken to the management of potential claims, with early investigation of incidents allowing information to be gathered whilst the incident is still fresh in the minds of the staff involved.

Incidents also can be reported verbally, sometimes using an answerphone system. This option is a useful adjunct to incident report forms, being particularly helpful when the workload is heavy and staff may balk at the completion of another form.

All incident reports should be reviewed on a daily basis to ensure that they are investigated promptly, with any necessary risk control measures being instigated as soon as possible. It is important that there is feedback to staff as to the outcome of the investigation into any incident they have reported, or in which they were involved. This encourages reporting of future incidents. The use of a computerized database facilitates the tracking of incidents, thus enabling any trends to be identified. In maternity units without their own risk manager, it is helpful if copies of forms submitted are sent also to a designated midwifery manager or supervisor of midwives. This allows him or her to have early knowledge of any incidents in which there are implications for midwifery practice.

Client satisfaction and complaints

An important source of information with regard to the quality of midwifery care is feedback from women and their families. In addition to unsolicited comments and complaints, this also can be obtained through the use of consumer satisfaction surveys.

From the risk management perspective, this feedback can be used to highlight areas of risk where the care received was sub-optimal or did not meet the client's expectations. It is important to differentiate between these two types of deficiencies in care. Whilst sub-optimal care may clearly put the woman and/or her baby at direct risk of harm, perceived failure to meet her expectations may be due to failures in communication between the woman and the midwifery (or other) staff caring for her. These are, in themselves, an important risk issue (see Chapter 2).

In addition, the psychological effects of outcomes that do not correlate with the woman's wishes or expectations have for some years been recognized as one of the possible triggers for the development of postnatal depression (Oakley and Chamberlain, 1981). More recent research has linked a woman's bad experience of childbirth with the subsequent development of post-traumatic stress disorder (Crompton, 1996).

Complaints, whether written or verbal, should be given equal priority with regard to their investigation. Each Trust should have a complaints procedure that complies with the guidance issued by the NHS Executive in EL(96)19. All complaints should be recorded, preferably on a computerized database that is linked to the databases used for managing clinical incidents and claims. This allows these to be cross-referenced, with early warning being given of potential claims. A prompt and full response to a complaint may prevent it from escalating into a claim, with the complainant seeking only an explanation of what went wrong, an apology if warranted, and reassurance that the same thing will not happen to someone else.

Clinical audit

In the context of the quality and effectiveness of care, clinical risk management and clinical audit are complementary systems, both of which lie at the heart of clinical governance. Aspects of Maxwell's quality framework of effectiveness, efficiency, appropriateness, acceptability, access and equity (Maxwell, 1984) are relevant to both, with the care provided being measured against agreed standards. Indeed, the use of a combination of these factors, together with the Donabedian classification of structure, process and outcome (Donabedian, 1986), provides a useful framework for both quality and risk assessments (Moss, 1995).

Clinical audit measures the effectiveness and appropriateness of the processes required to achieve specific outcomes. The results of the audit process highlight any deficiencies where practice parameters need to be changed; examples of this in maternity care are the *Confidential Enquiries into Maternal Deaths*, and the *Confidential Enquiries into Stillbirths and Deaths in Infancy* (CESDI). At a local level, an example is the regular, multidisciplinary audit meetings of midwives, obstetricians and paediatricians held in the majority of maternity units. These are used to discuss the management of specific cases where either the outcome has been poor, or it is considered that there are lessons to be learned from that particular case.

These examples demonstrate the overlap between clinical audit and risk management, and the consequent importance of good communication between the two departments. The audit findings become a risk management tool by identifying particular risks. These are then targeted through the risk management process, which aims to introduce agreed changes in practice to control these risks, thus completing the audit cycle. The audit is then repeated to determine whether the control measures have been successful.

Risk analysis

Once risks have been identified, the next step in the risk management process is to analyse them. The analysis findings will indicate what risk control measures are required, and will help determine the priority these should be given.

Probability and severity of outcome

Probability (or likelihood) and severity are the two main variables considered. Analysis of these two aspects of the risks identified can be used to prioritize the implementation of risk control measures, with those ranked as high risk being addressed first.

In industry, where the risk management process originated, the analysis of these factors would be based largely on hard, statistical data derived from previous performance. In clinical risk management this is more difficult because, although the rate of clinical incidents as a whole can be predicted (e.g. a study in one maternity unit showed 14 per cent of all deliveries had been affected by adverse events – O'Connor and Beard, 1996), these are usually the result of a combination of several factors, which may differ from incident to incident. The use of computerized databases for logging clinical incidents does allow tracking and trending of incidents to be undertaken, which can assist with the estimation of probability and severity. However, this remains a somewhat subjective exercise.

For practical purposes, one of the simplest methods is to devise a prioritization table (Table 8.3) based on the formula:

Risk = Severity of outcome × Probability of outcome.

The outcomes are divided into categories, which are given numerical values. The two values are multiplied, which gives the degree of risk exposure. In the example given (see Table 8.3), if the result is multiplied by five the risk exposure can be expressed in percentage terms.

It is important that the criteria for the various categories are agreed before the analysis is undertaken so that these are applied consistently. In the example given below the probability categories have been defined, but those relating to severity would need to be made explicit. These outcomes could be considered under the following headings:

- Staff injury (including length of time off work)
- Patient injury (including prolonged inpatient stay, increased morbidity)
- Financial loss to patient/staff

Table 8.3 Prioritization of risk outcomes

	Value
Severity rating:	
Catastrophic	5
Severe	4
Moderate	3
Low	2
Insignificant	1
Probability rating:	
Likely to occur at any time	4
Will probably occur in time	3
May occur in time	2
Unlikely to occur	1

- Financial loss to the Trust (e.g. cost of staff absence, damage to or loss of facilities, costs of subsequent litigation)
- Effect on the reputation of the Trust.

Other factors need to be considered when compiling a risk management action plan. These include:

- Ease of implementation
- Cost of implementation
- Timescale.

Safecode, which is a risk management tool developed for the NHS, takes this process a stage further by analysing the risk reduction potential and the benefit rating. The risk reduction potential (RRP) is the reduction in the risk rating (equates to the level of risk) following the implementation of risk control measures, with the benefit rating being the RRP plus any additional benefits that result from the risk control measures. The subsequent report, based on the risk analysis, can therefore identify the risks, indicate their probability and severity, and demonstrate the likely effect of the proposed risk control measures. A cost–benefit analysis can then be undertaken to inform further the prioritization exercise.

Fault tree analysis

This is a diagrammatic representation of the root causes underlying a particular risk situation (Figure 8.4). It demonstrates the possible chain of events leading to systems failures, whether these are due to human factors (see below) or to mechanical failure. It may be used in conjunction with a flow chart, which illustrates the process being undertaken. Whilst very comprehensive, it would not be practicable to undertake such analysis for all the risks identified. Nevertheless it is a useful tool, which may be needed when addressing more complex and intractable risks. Additionally, it can be used to calculate probability or frequency of occurrence if quantitative data relevant to the particular risk path are available. This is more relevant to non-clinical risks.

Human factors

The analysis of a clinical incident or near miss usually reveals this to be the result of several individual factors that combined to cause the incident. If the underlying causes are not addressed, a different combination of such factors could result in the occurrence of another incident. The human factors approach concentrates on the underlying organizational systems that are the root cause of such incidents, rather than on the individual midwife or other member of staff directly involved. This approach to risk management is being used increasingly, in conjunction with an incident reporting system, as a psychological tool with which to analyse the incidents reported (Vincent *et al.*, 1998).

The causation pathway for an incident has been described (Reason, 1995), with the latent factors as the root cause influencing the working conditions, which in turn give rise to the predisposing factors leading to the errors or violations (known as active failures) that are the direct cause of the incident

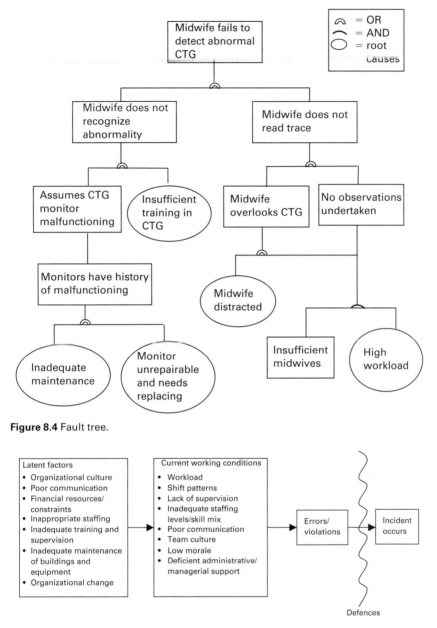

Figure 8.4 Fault tree.

Figure 8.5 Human factors model of clinical incident pathway.

(Figure 8.5). For an incident to occur, these have to overcome any defences or barriers in place (e.g. alarm systems, guidelines).

The analysis of causes needs to examine the following areas:

- Team factors (e.g. team culture, openness, communication)
- Task factors (e.g. equipment maintenance)

Table 8.4 Factors predisposing to errors and violations

Errors	Violations
High workload	Manager–staff conflict
Inadequate knowledge, ability or experience	Low morale
Stressful environment	Poor supervision
Inadequate supervision/training	Group norms condone actions
Mental state	Time pressure
Change	Ambiguous or meaningless rules

- Situational factors (e.g. time shortage, unfamiliarity with task, information overload)
- Organizational factors (e.g. incompatible goals, poor operating procedures, understaffing, high workload, inadequate training).

Although each member of staff is an individual, it has been observed that some factors predispose towards errors, with violations possibly having different or additional underlying causes (Table 8.4). Errors include unsafe acts and omissions due to memory lapses and 'honest' mistakes; violations are deliberate deviations from required standards, procedures or working practices. These are not necessarily malicious, and may take the form of 'cutting corners' to save time. The type of incident reported therefore may indicate which factors should be examined first.

As well as being used reactively to analyse the causes of clinical incidents, the human factors approach can be employed proactively to identify the presence of specified risk factors before any incident has occurred. Research has identified a checklist of background factors that can be used in conjunction with face-to-face interviews with staff as part of the risk identification process (Stanhope *et al.*, 1997).

References

Alexander, S. and Keirse, M. J. N. C. (1989). Formal risk scoring during pregnancy. In: *Effective Care in Pregnancy and Childbirth*, Vol. 1, pp. 345–65. Oxford University Press.

Capstick, B. (1994). Risk management in obstetrics. In: *Safe Practice in Obstetrics and Gynaecology* (R. V. Clements, ed.), pp. 405–16. Churchill Livingstone.

Clinical Negligence Scheme for Trusts (1999). *Clinical Risk Management Standards*. NHSLA.

Crompton, J. (1996). Post-traumatic stress disorder and childbirth. *Br. J. Midwifery*, **4(6)**, 290–94.

Dineen, M. (1996). Clinical risk management – a pragmatic approach., *Br. J. Midwifery*, **4(11)**, 586–9.

Donabedian, A. (1986). Evaluating the quality of medical care. *Millband Memorial Fund Q.*, **64(3)**, 166–206.

Genn, H. (1995). Supporting staff involved in litigation. In: *Clinical Risk Management* (C. Vincent, ed.), pp. 453–72. BMJ Publishing Group.

Maxwell, R. (1984). Quality assessment in health. *Br. Med. J.*, **288**, 1470–72.

Miller, S. (1999). Critical incidences and the value of reflective thinking. *Br. J. Midwifery*, **7(1)**, 19–22.

Moss, F. (1995). Risk management and quality of care. In: *Clinical Risk Management* (C. Vincent, ed.), pp. 88–102. BMJ Publishing Group.

NHSME (1993). *Risk Management in the NHS*, pp. 1–2. DoH.

Oakley, A. and Chamberlain, G, (1981) Medical and social factors in postpartum depression. *J. Obstet. Gynaecol.*, **1**, 182–7.

O'Connor, A. M. and Beard, R. W. (1996). Risk management – what is it and how does it work? *MIDIRS Midwifery Digest*, **6(1)**, 61–4.

Reason, J. (1995). Understanding adverse events: human factors. In: *Clinical Risk Management* (C. Vincent, ed.), pp. 31–54. BMJ Publishing Group.

Royal College of Obstetricians and Gynaecologists and Royal College of Midwives (1999). *Towards Safer Childbirth: Minimum Standards for the Organisation of Labour Wards*. RCOG Press.

Smith, J. A. and Mitchell, S. (1996). Debriefing after childbirth: a tool for effective risk management. *Br. J. Midwifery*, **4(11)**, 581–6.

Stanhope, N., Vincent, C., Taylor-Adams, S. *et al*. (1997). Applying human factors methods to clinical risk management in obstetrics. *Br. J. Obstet. Gynaecol.*, **104**, 1225–32.

Vincent, C. (1995). Caring for patients harmed by treatment. In: *Clinical Risk Management* (C. Vincent, ed.), pp. 433–52. BMJ Publishing Group.

Vincent, C. (1997). Risk, safety and the dark side of quality. *Br. Med. J.*, **314**, 1775–6.

Vincent, C., Taylor-Adams, S. and Stanhope, N. (1998). Framework for analysing risk and safety in clinical medicine. *Br. Med. J.*, **316**, 1154–7.

Welsh Risk Pool (1999). *Risk Management Standards*.

Wilson, J. H. (1999) Clinical Risk Modification: A Route to Clinical Governance. Butterworth–Heinemann.

9

The consumer view

Mary Nolan

Introduction

Today, it is likely that a minimum of four people are present at the birth of a child; these are the mother and her baby, the mother's chosen support person – often the father of her child – and the midwife, whose job it is to care for all three. All of these people are hoping for a satisfactory outcome, which both parents and midwives define as a 'perfect healthy baby' and a 'satisfying experience' (Proctor, 1998). The phrase 'ecological birth' has been used to describe an event that leaves all participants whole in body and mind. Birth should do no harm to anyone involved in the experience.

With the perinatal mortality rate in the UK at its lowest ever, women do not expect to lose their baby at or around birth. Nor do they expect to be seriously injured or die themselves as a result of childbearing. This situation does not, of course, apply in less privileged parts of the world, where the vast majority of the half a million women who do die each year as a result of childbearing are to be found. As western women's basic needs for safety around birth are increasingly met, their desire to achieve mental health in relation to childbearing becomes more prominent (*cf.* Maslow's hierarchy of needs; Maslow, 1968). This does not indicate, as an obstetrician lecturing an audience of antenatal teachers once commented, that women in this country are so 'spoiled' that all they have left to worry about are the most trivial details of care, but rather a natural and healthy progression in women's attempt to fulfil every facet of their humanity.

It is surely the aim, whether as midwives or volunteers working to make the maternity service more responsive to the needs of women and their families, to ensure that not only the physical health of childbearing women but also their mental health is not put at risk. The work of Oakley (1980) on the links between what happens to a woman during childbirth and her postnatal mood suggests at a high level of significance that 'dissatisfaction with birth management' is related to postnatal depression. Oakley also found that 'low self-image as a mother' which results from a woman's perception that she was out of control during labour is significantly related to poor feelings for the baby. She concluded, therefore, that the experience of labour is critical in shaping the early relationship between a mother and her child. The importance of women surviving labour with intact self-esteem has also been highlighted by Sosa *et al.* (1980) and Kennell and Klaus (1991). These authors suggest that by helping the woman to maximize her own resources for coping with contractions, by praising her and keeping her fully informed about and involved in decisions regarding pain relief, instrumental delivery and the condition of her baby, her self-esteem will be enhanced and thereby her ability to parent her new-born child.

Every woman's needs

In 1993 the Conservative Government published a seminal report on the maternity services entitled *Changing Childbirth*, which summarized and offered guidance to healthcare professionals on what it is that women find satisfying about their care. The Report's conclusions were encapsulated in its much repeated but nonetheless vital first principle of good care (DoH, p. 8):

The woman must be the focus of maternity care. She should be able to feel that she is in control of what is happening to her and able to make decisions about her care, based on her needs, having discussed matters fully with the professionals involved.

Whether *Changing Childbirth* was truly a blueprint for a maternity service that would reflect the aspirations of a diverse nation was questioned by some, who pointed out that the women who had given evidence to the Expert Maternity Group were, on the whole, articulate activists working for middle-class organizations such as the National Childbirth Trust and the Association for Improvement in the Maternity Services. However, the work of Green *et al.* (1988) refutes the suggestion that women from different socio-demographic groups have radically different needs. This research described two stereotypes of child-bearing women, one the 'well-educated, middle-class, NCT type' and the other the 'uneducated, working-class woman', and found that whilst a greater number of highly educated women wanted control over decision-making, 65 per cent of the least educated women (who had left school at 16) wanted at least to have issues discussed with them. Not a single woman in the sample of 825 said that she definitely did not want to be in control of what was done to her by staff, and the vast majority of women of all educational levels either wanted control 'very much' or would 'quite like' to be in control of what doctors and midwives did to them during labour. Less educated women were as keen as those more highly educated to avoid medical forms of pain relief, and were not less prone to depression after childbirth. The authors concluded from their data that the stereotypes of the middle-class NCT type who has unrealistically high expectations of childbirth and of the uneducated working class woman who refuses to take any responsibility for informing herself could not be supported. Grant's work (1987) and the 1990 NAHAT Report confirm that black and ethnic minority women want the same things from the maternity service as do women from the majority white culture. All groups of women want a flexible service in which individual wishes are respected, waiting times are kept to a minimum, privacy is safeguarded, information is readily available, and communication is open and courteous (Schott and Henley, 1996):

In general, it is not different services, but more flexible and responsive services that are needed to ensure equal access. Providing different services to different communities on the basis of narrow definitions of their cultures, customs and traditions can simply result in the creation of new stereotypes and is usually not necessary.

Reducing the risks: information and informed consent

In her study of survivors of incest, Parratt (1994) identified the factors that help an abused woman to experience birth positively:

- Trust in her birth attendants, which is promoted by continuity of care and carer from the antenatal period through to the postnatal
- Privacy during labour
- Being kept informed
- Being in control of decisions regarding her care and interventions during labour.

This study focused on the most vulnerable women, but it is self-evident that a system that protects and empowers the least privileged will also accommodate the welfare of the more privileged.

All women want information about their care and to be in control of what is happening to them. Information and control are closely linked because information is power, and when professionals withhold information they pre-empt control and jurisdiction on the part of their clients (Tagliacozzo and Mauksch, 1979). It is impossible to operationalize the concept of 'informed choice' unless consumers are knowledgeable (Qureshi *et al.*, 1996). The study by Green *et al.* (1988) concluded that 'the majority of women wanted to know as much as possible about what might happen in labour'. Knowing what questions to ask (which comes from already being well informed) enables further information to be obtained. The Finnish Family Competence Study (Rautava *et al.*, 1991) noted that women with low levels of knowledge did not question the professional care they received, and were 'disappointed' and 'shocked' by their childbirth experiences. Women with high knowledge 'asked questions significantly more often on the postnatal ward than low knowledge mothers'.

In an editorial for the *British Journal of Midwifery*, Schott (1994) commented that not only does acquiring research-based information put women in a better position to make informed choices, but it also enables them 'to develop confidence and self-esteem'. In Cahill and Mathis' research (1990), primiparous women commented that 'information helped to reduce feelings of helplessness about labour and childbirth'. Some groups of women have been found to lack very basic knowledge about pregnancy and childbirth. Shapiro *et al.* (1983) noted that women from disadvantaged social groups needed information on a wide range of topics, but that the lower their social group, the less likely they were to obtain the information they wanted. Comerford *et al.* (1991) carried out a study of 211 pregnant women living in an inner city, and found that almost half did not know how many weeks constituted a normal pregnancy and a third were unaware that premature babies can have respiratory problems. Poverty reduces access to education and access to health services because women have neither the confidence nor the ability to use the services to their own advantage. Health professionals may find it difficult to communicate with disadvantaged women (Fleissig, 1993), yet it is these women who are most at risk of losing their baby at or around birth, diminished self-esteem as a result of their childbearing experiences, and depression associated with social isolation (Chadwick, 1994).

Symon (1998) has pointed to the link between inadequate information giving and litigation. An independent midwife, quoted in his analysis of why people sue, comments:

The majority of people who sue, sue to get more information, to find out what actually happened

and Symon concludes that where communication and trust between service users and providers fail, 'the possibility of dissatisfaction (whether or not there has been a poor clinical outcome) is much greater'.

Reducing the risks: power in the midwife–mother encounter

While there is much evidence to support the claim that women, whether having their first or subsequent babies, and of whatever educational level or social group, wish to have information in order to feel more in control, it is also clear that often they do not ask for it (Kirke 1980). Proctor's study (1998) states:

Antenatal care was characterized primarily by a need for information, understanding and reassurance ... The importance of being offered information was mentioned frequently by women, particularly concerning their anxiety in not knowing what to ask about antenatal procedures or tests. Many did not feel confident asking for advice because they perceived the staff to be too busy to spend time with them.

Perkins (1991) suggests that women don't ask for the type of care they want and therefore, not surprisingly, often don't get it. In her opinion, women are not used to defining their needs and are insufficiently assertive in voicing them. They may also have no expectations that the service will be interested in them. It is important to recognize that the medicalization of childbirth and the role of 'patient' which that enforces makes it very difficult for women to obtain information upon which to base choices.

In the traditional encounter between a doctor and patient, the doctor is dominant and the patient accepts (generally willingly) a subordinate position. The lower the social class of the patient, the more exaggerated these roles become. Patients try hard to adjust their behaviour to meet the expectations of health professional staff. This often means not asking for too much information, first because staff are busy and it is inconsiderate to impose on their time, and secondly because any questioning might be seen as a lack of confidence in their expertise (Tagliacozzo and Mauksch, 1979). The author's own experience of teaching assertiveness in antenatal classes fully bears out the frequently noted unwillingness on the part of the best-educated and most articulate people to ask questions of medical and midwifery staff for fear of being considered 'an awkward customer'. Pregnant women have, for the most part, wholeheartedly taken on the role of patient. Machin and Scamell (1997) discuss the influence of the hospital environment on labouring women:

In this place, the women felt bewildered and it would seem the authority of the metaphor of science and medicine, and the need to pass over the boundary to the safety of the white coats and medication, became overwhelming.

Many studies (Mander, 1993; Bluff and Holloway, 1994; Floyd, 1995) have identified the shift in thinking that is required if health carers are really to grasp the need to share information fully with women. Ralston (1994) observes that:

> *Many professionals have an innate attitude of superiority and a reluctance to divulge more than the minimum amount of information when dealing with clients.*

The interface between women's and midwives' autonomy is not yet properly explored, and whilst professionals may fear the loss of control entailed in divulging information, women may not understand that making their own choices must involve acceptance of responsibility for the outcome of those choices. The education of consumers of health care in a market-driven health service is yet in its infancy, and is one of the key elements that will allow health professionals to share the responsibility for the outcomes of care and treatment with their clients (Leavey *et al.*, 1989).

Reducing the risks: accessible and relevant information

Some studies have provided insights into what kind of information women require, when they require it and how it should be delivered. Ley (1988) has identified three problems that lead to failure to communicate effectively with women. These are:

1. Presenting information in a way that is too difficult for the woman to understand
2. Failing to appreciate that women may not have even an elementary knowledge of the anatomy and physiology of reproduction
3. Not identifying the 'old wives' tales' that mould women's expectations of childbearing.

Women want a constant supply of information, even when it might be considered that they are least able to absorb it. Fleissig (1993) notes that women need to be kept informed throughout labour about how the birth is progressing, and Berg *et al.* (1996) remark that:

> *Even in emergency situations, the women wanted the staff to stop for just a second and communicate with them. Eye contact and explanation of the reason for interventions, followed by a moment of thinking, were desired in order to maintain control and feel part of the birthing process.*

Schott (1994) touches on the importance of listening before giving information. Information needs to be tailored to an individual's needs, and unless the woman is allowed time to think about what the key issues are for her personally it will not be possible for carers to identify the most useful information for her and help her apply it to her particular situation.

The role of antenatal classes – realism in adult education

The education of adults is not about engineering 'learner consent to take the actions favoured by the educator' (Mezirow, 1983). Adult learners are self-directing and need to grow in independence, not in dependency on the teacher.

This is especially true of antenatal education, where adult learners are seeking help to prepare for the most responsible job they will ever undertake in their lives – parenthood. Education is rarely, if ever, about advice-giving; rather, according to Rogers (1996, p. 18), teachers:

> ... *seek to bring the student participants into contact with the primary material and leave them free to use it themselves.*

The environment of the antenatal class is therefore one in which parents-to-be and their chosen support people build on the information they already have about giving birth and caring for young children, validate their feelings by sharing them with others, work out practical approaches to the challenges of early parenting, and learn (through the co-operation modelled in the class) about the importance of parent-to-parent support.

There is an extensive literature on antenatal education, highlighting in particular topics that women feel are insufficiently well covered in classes. These include deviations from the normal course of labour, such as assisted deliveries and Caesarean sections (Hillan, 1992); babies who are stillborn, severely disabled or seriously ill (Fleissig, 1993); and postnatal issues such as mental health after the birth and basic babycare skills (Gould, 1986; McKay and Yager Smith, 1993). Above all, parents seek a realistic portrayal of birth and early parenthood.

In the 1950s, the American doctor and psychologist Irving Janis looked at how his patients coped with major surgery. He found that the patients who recovered most speedily from their operations were those who had had realistic expectations beforehand, based on good quality information, of what the surgery would involve. Janis (1958, p. 376–7) described the process these patients had been through prior to surgery as 'the anticipatory work of worrying', and concluded that:

> *The more thorough the work of worrying, the more adequate the subsequent adjustment to any given type of danger or deprivation ... This mental activity leads to action and mastery of the threat situation.*

Women can be helped to meet the challenges of childbirth only if they are prepared for the realities of what they will or may experience. The work of Melzack (1984) demonstrates that mothers whose expectations of labour are unrealistic experience worse pain than mothers with more realistic expectations. If women build up realistic expectations in the antenatal period, the possibilities of disappointment, guilt and anger are diminished. Enabling women and their families to do the anticipatory work of worrying may enable them to have more control over labour and protect their mental health, whatever the outcome of birth. Janis suggests that preparation for a major and possibly distressing life event should be approached in a variety of ways. First, he recommends that (Janis, 1958):

> *The more precisely every potentially frightening perceptual experience is described, the lower the chances that the given experience will have a traumatizing effect.*

The important word here is 'perceptual'. Janis suggests that patients do not need detailed technical accounts of medical procedures, but they do need to learn about and try to imagine the sensory experiences they will go through and how

they might respond emotionally. In terms of childbirth education, this means looking at labour from the parents' point of view. Parents do not need to know how the surgeon carries out a Caesarean, but it is helpful for them to know that having a Caesarean under spinal is not sensation-free; as one woman said, 'it feels as if someone is doing the washing-up in your tummy!'.

Janis (1958) considers that patients can maintain 'active control' if they practise 'various anticipatory thought sequences' which will later ward off feelings of helplessness in the presence of fear-provoking stimuli. Women need to be given the opportunity in their antenatal classes to think through situations that might arise during labour and to develop skills for participating in decision-making around their own care. They need to learn the questions that underpin informed consent or informed refusal:

- What are the benefits of doing this?
- What might be the drawbacks?
- Are there any alternatives?
- What will happen if we do nothing?
- How long do we have to make up our minds about this?

Nolan's research (1997) into the effectiveness of antenatal education compared classes provided by the National Childbirth Trust and classes provided by midwives working in the NHS and concluded that, whichever kind parents had attended, they wanted much more information about practical postnatal issues. After they had completed their classes, parents' evaluation forms typically included such comments as:

> I would have liked more on coping with practical things e.g. bathing baby once baby comes home.

> What about recommended ointments, lotions, nappies etc.?

> Some comments about postnatal care, please – feeding, illness, bathing.

This theme became even stronger in the postnatal period, when parents were asked to reflect on their classes in the light of their lived experience of caring for their babies (taken from Nolan 1997):

> Classes should talk about common changes in babies, e.g. cradle cap, milk spots, wind, colic, etc. More information about this kind of thing – bathing and how often.

> Much more needed on practicalities after the birth – feeding, winding, typical medical problems etc.

Salamm (1995) notes how useful it is for pregnant women to have contact with mothers and their infants to learn from them how to care for babies. Inviting new parents and their babies to visit the antenatal class can raise many questions in pregnant parents' minds that they would not otherwise have thought of, and enables them to consider coping strategies that other people have found useful in making the transition to parenthood.

There is a strong argument for covering the very difficult issues of stillbirth, cot death, disability and prematurity in antenatal classes. Surprisingly often, parents will raise these topics themselves, seeking to have their anxieties validated by sharing them with others. Childbirth educators need to try to re-establish the understanding and acceptance, which have been lost over the years, that birth and death and birth and illness are sometimes closely related. Acceptance of adverse birth outcomes has been lost, first because infant mortality rates in this country have been very low for several decades; and secondly because government and health professionals have led women to believe that if they give birth in hospital under medical management, the safety and health of their babies will be guaranteed. To collude in such wrong ideas does neither parents nor health professionals any service; from unrealistic expectations spring litigation and depression.

Antenatal care for special parents: avoiding prejudice and identifying needs

Special consideration needs to be given to providing relevant antenatal education and care for parents with special needs, such as those who are disabled, those who speak English with difficulty, those with learning difficulties, those from ethnic minority groups, and very young parents. Education will be neither appropriate nor sensitive if the people who deliver it have not explored their own prejudices beforehand so that they can avoid the dangers of stereotyping. In the case of disabled people, typical stereotypes imposed by able-bodied people include (based on Campion and Jain, 1990):

- Disabled people don't have normal intelligence
- Disabled people are dependent
- A disabled person is an ill person
- All disabled women have to give birth by Caesarean
- The child of a disabled person is at risk
- A disabled person cannot be a proper parent.

Prejudice in educators negates teaching skills and denies parents learning opportunities. Beyond prejudice, useful learning opportunities for all groups of people can be identified. These include the following, which have been found by disabled parents to be helpful, and are relevant also to parents with other kinds of special needs (based on McEwan Carty *et al.*, 1990):

- A guided tour round the hospital where their baby is to be born, to familiarize themselves with the environment
- Talking to the staff who will care for them about their needs
- Being put in touch with other parents who share their special needs
- Being introduced to organizers of local mother and baby groups – isolation postnatally is a real problem for these parents
- Being put in touch with organizations with specialist knowledge of their situation
- Having individual attention, both antenatally and postnatally, to learn about infant feeding
- Seeing pictures of parents like themselves and their children in antenatal classes.

Research suggests that disabled women rely more on lay sources for guidance about baby care and equipment than they do on health professionals.

Birth plans and support in labour

Anecdotal evidence would suggest that midwives are unsure about the useful-ness of birth plans, fearing that by virtue of having written down what they would like for their labours, women are more likely to be disappointed if things do not go according to plan. The author's own experience suggests that many parents are anxious that a birth plan might be seen by their midwife as an unwelcome attempt to tell him or her what to do, or that it might limit the parents' flexibility to make on-the-spot decisions. Such anxieties are recognized by the National Childbirth Trust's leaflet *Making a Birth Plan* (NCT, 1997, p. 14), which reads:

> *Your midwife will try to help you achieve the kind of labour and birth you want. However, it is impossible for anyone to predict what your labour will be like, or how you will feel. Write your birth plan so that your midwife knows you are prepared to be flexible. Show that you know you may want to change your mind about some things.*

It is, of course, no use encouraging women to make birth plans if the support they will need on the labour ward to enable them to realize their wishes is not available. Some hospitals provide women with tick-box birth plans that ask them to indicate whether they want to be mobile during labour and what kind of pain relief they would prefer, including the option to do without pharmacological analgesia. However, women are only likely to remain active in labour and to use their own resources for coping with pain if they have continuous and sensitive support to enable them to achieve those ideals. They will naturally be disap-pointed if the assistance given by the midwife seems to be to help them to choose between pethidine or an epidural rather than to help them remain upright and focused on the breathing techniques they have learned in antenatal classes. Shearer (1990) identifies the yawning chasm that sometimes opens up between a woman's birth plan and her experience on the delivery suite:

> *Bedside practices can make prenatal education appear to be effective, or to have made no difference, or to have actually caused harm to patients. Obstetric staff do quickly ascertain the goals of patients admitted in labor and the goals of their prenatal classes. The staff have their own feelings about various classes, consciously or not. Usually, they have discussed how much they will co-operate with parents' wishes and which of their goals to promote, downgrade or ignore.*

Women who receive optimum support during labour are unlikely to be dissatis-fied with their birth experience, whatever its outcome. One category of support is information giving, which has been dealt with at length in this chapter. However, there are at least two further categories: emotional support – 'attach-ing, reassuring, giving the feeling that one is able to rely on or confide in a person, giving the feeling that one is cared about'; and tangible support – 'direct aid, such as taking care of someone' (Bryanton *et al.*, 1993). Research carried out in America has suggested that midwives are relatively unavailable to provide emotional and tangible support, with the proportion of time they spend in supportive versus all other activities being 9.9 per cent (McNiven *et al.*, 1992). The importance of one-to-one support for women in labour has been well established since the early 1980s. The seminal study is that of Sosa *et al.* (1980), which was carried out at the Social Security Hospital in Guatemala City, where it was the policy not to allow women to be attended by any companion of their choice during labour. The study randomly assigned 20 primiparous women to a control group who received the normal care provided by the hospital – namely intermittent visits from a midwife during the first stage, and continuous attention during the second and third – and 20 to an experimental group who received the same care but also the support of an untrained lay woman who remained with them from admission to delivery. The randomization process itself was illuminating in that 103 mothers had to be admitted to the control group but only 33 to the experimental group in order to obtain 20 in each group who achieved uncomplicated deliveries. Twenty-six per cent of the mothers in the control group had a Caesarean, but only 6 per cent of those in the experimental group. Augmentation of labour was carried out in 16 per cent of control group mothers but only 2 per cent of experimental group mothers. Most remarkable of all, the women who received the continuous support of another woman delivered their babies in approximately 8 hours as opposed to the 19 hours achieved by the unsupported women. In the postnatal period, the research-ers observed that the women in the experimental group stroked their babies and talked to them more frequently than the women who had had standard care during labour.

This famous study has been repeated in hospitals all over the world, including the United States (Kennell and Klaus, 1991) and South Africa (Hofmeyr *et al.*, 1991). The National Maternity Hospital in Dublin has made it the cornerstone of its policy of active management that each woman in labour should be supported by a midwife who stays with her from the moment she comes into hospital to after she has had her baby. Klaus *et al.* (1993, p. 98) comment:

The active management of labor has spread to many parts of Europe. Unfortunately, in most hospitals, the one-to-one nursing component has been left out. These hospitals have not appreciated the importance of this continuous care in easing and shortening labour ... In the National Maternity Hospital in Dublin, birthing is women's work. Women caring for women continue an age-old tradition. The midwife practises her craft with skill, caring and intuitive and experienced knowledge.

The experience of Michel Odent at his hospital in Pithiviers, France, also points to the fact that intervention rates can be reduced to a minimum and women's satisfaction with giving birth and their mental health in the postnatal period maximized when quality support is made available to them in labour (Odent, 1994). It should be remembered that fathers have never been shown to be as effective in supporting women in labour as have other women, and that they may be as much in need of support themselves as their partners are (Niven, 1985; Chalmers and Wolman, 1993).

The escalation in intervention during labour and birth does not promote women's self-esteem, and nor does it guarantee the physical wellbeing of the mother and her baby. More than 20 years ago, Chard and Richards (1977, p. 35) pointed to the hazards of the 'new obstetrics', commenting:

As these interventions are applied to an increasingly large proportion of the obstetric and fetal population, a threshold will inevitably be reached beyond which the marginal risks of the procedures will outweigh the marginal benefits.

It would appear that one way of reducing mass intervention in labour and the physical and emotional risks associated with it is to provide each labouring woman with one-to-one support from another woman. The word often used for such a support person is 'doula', a Greek word that refers to an experienced woman who guides and assists a new mother in childbirth and infant care. Many midwives would like to be doulas, but are prevented by shortages of staff, the demands of paperwork, and the obligation to conform to hospital protocols which distract them from responding to the minute-by-minute changes in the needs of the labouring woman. Recognizing this gap in support, some UK hospitals are already welcoming lay-women who volunteer their services to support mothers who have no partner or friend to be with them during labour (Nolan, 1995). The financial implications of bringing doulas into delivery suites could be substantial – Wagner (1994) calculated that if the Caesarean rate in the USA were to fall from 24 per cent to 15 per cent, a saving of $1000 million a year would be achieved. The emotional implications in terms of increasing women's satisfaction with birth and enhancing their early relationship with their newborn infants could be even more substantial.

Reducing the risks: finding out what women want

This chapter has touched upon some of the critical areas for midwives to consider in order to minimize the risk that the experience of birth might put in jeopardy the physical or mental health of any of those present. These areas include information giving, the interface between midwives' and mothers' autonomy, education to facilitate informed consent or refusal, realistic preparation of women in the antenatal period for normal and unexpected birth outcomes, and support in labour. Further progress can be made in the direction of a maternity service that is truly responsive to the needs of women when women themselves become involved in defining the agenda for research, in gathering and analysing data, and in disseminating results throughout their communities. Entwistle *et al.* (1998) argue the importance of paying greater attention to lay perspectives in order to improve the quality of research:

> *Patients may also have important insights that researchers may overlook – insights into things that cause problems for patients, or the types of technology and outcomes that patients value or are concerned about ... Lay involvement in generating knowledge may increase the perceived relevance and acceptance of findings. The inclusion of lay perspectives may therefore lead to research findings being more fully implemented.*

User involvement in medical audit is increasingly being seen not merely as desirable but as essential both to assist healthcare professionals in remaining focused on the issues that are important to clients, and also to protect scarce financial resources (Joule, 1992, p. 10):

> *Users are less likely to demand ineffective (though 'fashionable') treatments or procedures if they are informed through involvement in the auditing process.*

If the evidence upon which practice is based is generated as a result of involving women at every stage of the research process, it seems probable that dissatisfaction with the care provided and consequent unhappiness on the part of women and their families and litigation against the maternity service can be avoided. When maternity care fully acknowledges the views of women, it will surely develop so as to ensure that every woman has the opportunity to:

- *Have a healthy and joyous birth experience for herself and her family, regardless of age or circumstances;*
- *Give birth as she wishes in an environment in which she feels nurtured and secure, and her emotional wellbeing, privacy, and personal preferences are respected;*
- *Have access to the full range of options for pregnancy, birth, and nurturing her baby, and to accurate information on all available birthing sites, caregivers, and practices;*
- *Receive accurate and up-to-date information about the benefits and risks of all procedures, drugs, and tests suggested for use during pregnancy, birth, and the postpartum period, with the rights to informed consent and informed refusal;*
- *Receive support for making informed choices about what is best for her and her baby based on individual values and beliefs.*

(Mother-Friendly Childbirth Initiative, 1996)

References

Berg, M., Lundgren, I., Hermansson, E. and Wahlberg V. (1996). Women's experience of the encounter with the midwife during childbirth. *Midwifery*, **12**, 11–15.

Bluff, R. and Holloway, I. (1994). 'They know best': women's perceptions of midwifery care during labour and childbirth. *Midwifery*, **10(3)**, 157–64.

Bryanton, J., Fraser-Davey, H. and Sullivan P. (1993). Women's perceptions of nursing support during labour. *J. Obstet. Gynecol. Neonatal Nursing*, **23(8)**, 638–43.

Cahill, J. M. and Mathis, D. M. (1990). Pretesting a childbirth handbook. *Birth*, **17(1)**, 39–42.

Campion, M. and Jain, (1990). *The Baby Challenge: A Handbook on Pregnancy for Women with a Physical Disability.* Tavistock Routledge.

Chadwick, J. (1994). Perinatal mortality and antenatal care. *Modern Midwife*, **4(9)**, 18–20.

Chalmers, B. and Wolman, W. (1993). Social support in labor – a selective review. *J. Psychosom. Obstet. Gynaecol.*, **14**, 1–15.

Chard T. and Richards M. (eds) (1977). *Benefits and Hazards of the New Obstetrics.* Spastics International Medical Publications.

Comerford, F. M., Damus, K. and Merkatz, I. (1991). What do pregnant women know about preventing pre-term birth? *J. Obstet. Gynaecol. Neonatal Nursing*, **20(2)**, 140–45.

Department of Health (1993). *Changing Childbirth*, Part 1. HMSO.

Entwistle, V. A., Renfrew, M. J., Yearley, S. *et al.* (1998). Lay perspectives: advantages for health research. *Br. Med. J.*, **316**, 463–6.

Fleissig, A. (1993). Are women given enough information by staff during labour and delivery? *Midwifery*, **9**, 70–75.

Floyd, L. (1995). Community midwives' views and experience of home birth. *Midwifery*, **11**, 3–10.

Gould, D. (1986). Locally organised antenatal classes and their effectiveness. *Nursing Times*, **82(45)**, 59–61.

Grant, J. (1987). Getting it right. *Medicine Soc.*, **13(2)**, 21–5.

Green, J. M., Coupland. V. A. and Kitzinger, J. V. (1988). *Great Expectations: A Prospective Study of Women's Expectations and Experiences of Childbirth.* Child Care Dev. Group, University of Cambridge.

Hillan, E. (1992). Issues in the delivery of midwifery care. *J. Adv. Nursing*, **17**, 274–8.

Hofmeyr, G. J., Nikodem, V. C., Wolman, W. L. *et al.* (1991). Companionship to modify the clinical birth environment: effects on progress and perceptions of labour, and breastfeeding. *Br. J. Obstet. Gynaecol.*, **98**, 756–64.

Janis, I. L. (1958). *Psychological Stress: Psychoanalytic and Behavioral Studies of Surgical Patients.* Academic Press.

Joule, N. (1992). *User Involvement in Medical Audit.* Greater London Association of Community Health Councils.

Kirke, P. N. (1980). Mothers' views of obstetric care. *Br. J. Obstet. Gynaecol.*, **87**, 1029–33.

Kennell, M. D. and Klaus, M. (1991), Continuous emotional support during labor in a US hospital. *J. Am. Med. Assoc.*, **265(17)**, 2197–201.

Klaus, M. H., Kennell, J. H. and Klaus, P. H. (1993). *Mothering the Mother.* Addison Wesley Publishing Co.

Leavey, R., Wilkin, D. and Metcalfe D. H. H. (1989). Consumerism and general practice. *Br. Med. J.*, **298**, 737–9.

Ley, (1988). *Communicating with Patients: Improving Communication, Satisfaction and Compliance.* Chapman and Hall.

Machin, D. and Scamell, M. (1997). The experience of labour: using ethnography to explore the irresistible nature of the biomedical metaphor during labour. *Midwifery*, **13(2)**, 78–84.

Mander, R. (1993). Autonomy in midwifery and maternity care. *Midwives Chronicle*, **106(1269)**, 369–74.

Maslow, A. H. (1968). *Toward a Psychology of Being*, 2nd edn. Van Nostrand Reinhold.

McEwan Carty E., Conine, T. and Hall, L. (1990). Comprehensive health promotion for the pregnant woman who is disabled. *J. Nurse-Midwifery*, **35(3)**, 134–6.

McKay, S. and Yager Smith, S. (1993). What are they talking about? Is something wrong? Information sharing during the second stage of labor. *Birth*, **20(3)**, 142–7.

McNiven, P., Hodnett, E. and O'Brien-Pallas, L. (1992). Supporting women in labor: a work sampling study of the activities of labor and delivery nurses. *Birth*, **19(1)**, 3–8.

Melzack, R. (1984). The myth of painless childbirth –the John F. Bonica lecture. *Pain*, **19**, 321–37.

Mezirow, J. (1983). A critical theory of adult learning and education. In: *Adult Learning and Education* (M. Tight, ed.), p. 135. Croom Helm.

Mother-Friendly Childbirth Initiative: The First Consensus Initiative of the Coalition for Improving Maternity Services (1996). Published in: *Int. J. Childbirth Ed.*, **13(2)**, 26–8 (copyright free).

National Association of Health Authorities and Trusts (1990). *Words about Action: Bulletin No. 2.* Maternity Services.

National Childbirth Trust/TESCO (1997). *Making a Birth Plan.* Book Production Consultants plc.

Niven, C. (1985). How helpful is the presence of the husband at childbirth? *J. Reprod. Infant Psychol.*, **3**, 45–53.

Nolan, M. (1995). Supporting women in labour – the role of the doula. *Modern Midwife*, **5(3)**, 12–15.

Nolan, M. (1997). Antenatal education – failing to educate for parenthood. *Br. J. Midwifery*, **5(1)**, 21–6.

Oakley, A. (1980). *Women Confined*, p. 142. Martin Robertson.

Odent, M. (1994). *Birth Reborn: What Childbirth Should Be.* Souvenir Press.

Parratt, J. (1994). The experience of childbirth for the survivors of incest. *Midwifery*, **10**, 26–39.

Perkins, E. R. (1991). What do women want? Asking consumers' views. Mable Liddiard Memorial Lecture. *Midwives' Chronicle*, **104(1247)**, 347–54.

Proctor, S. (1998). What determines quality in maternity care? Comparing the perceptions of childbearing women and midwives. *Birth*, **25(2)**, 85–93.

Qureshi, N. S., Schofield, G., Papaioannou, S. *et al.* (1996). Parentcraft classes: do they affect outcome in childbirth? *J. Obstet. Gynaecol.*, **1(6)**, 358–61.

Ralston, R. (1994). How much choice do women really have in relation to their care? *Br. J. Midwifery*, **2(9)**, 453–6.

Rautava, P., Erkkola, R. and Sillanpaa, M. (1991). The outcome and experiences of first pregnancy in relation to the mother's childbirth knowledge: the Finnish Family Competence Study. *J. Adv. Nursing*, **16**, 1226–32.

Rogers, A. (1996). *Teaching Adults*. Open University Press.

Salamm, C. M. (1995). Mothers' perceptions of infant care and self-care competence after early postpartum discharge. *Birth*, **10(2)**, 30–39.

Schott, J. (1994). The importance of encouraging women to think for themselves. *Br. J. Midwifery*, **2(1)**, 3–4.

Schott, J. and Henley, A. (1996). *Culture, Religion and Childbearing in a Multiracial Society*. Butterworth-Heinemann.

Shapiro, M. C., Najman, J. M., Chang, A. *et al.* (1983). Information, control and the exercise of power in the obstetrical encounter. *Social Sci. Med.*, **17(3)**, 139–46.

Shearer, M. (1990). Effects of prenatal education depend on the attitudes and practices of obstetric caregivers. *Birth*, **17(2)**, 73–4.

Sosa, M. D., Kennell, J., Klaus, M. *et al.* (1980). The effect of a supportive companion on perinatal problems, length of labor, and mother–infant interaction. *N. Engl. J. Med.*, **303(11)**, 597–600.

Symon, A. (1998). Why do people sue? *Br. J. Midwifery*, **6(6)**, 395–8.

Tagliacozzo, D. and Mauksch, H. O. (1979). The patient's view of the patient's role. In: *Patients, Physicians and Illness: A Sourcebook in Behavioral Science and Health*, 3rd edn (E. Gartly Jaco, ed.), pp. 185–99. The Free Press.

Wagner, M. (1994). *Pursuing the Birth Machine: The Search for Appropriate Birth Technology*. ACE Graphics.

10

The victims of midwifery accidents

Liz Thomas and Georgina Tansley

Introduction

When the issue of the rise in costs associated with medical litigation is being discussed, attention is frequently focused on two areas: the increasingly litigious nature of our society, and a significant rise in patients' expectations of health care and its outcomes. Whilst there is certainly an element of truth in this rather crude analysis, it diverts attention away from the underlying reality that medical accidents or adverse clinical events are a greatly underestimated reality in healthcare provision.

Studies in both the USA and Australia have established that adverse events (defined as unintended injuries to patients caused by medical management) represent a significant problem within modern health care. In the American Harvard study (Brennan *et al.*, 1991), 30 121 randomly selected records from 51 acute care hospitals in New York State were reviewed. Adverse events occurred in 3.7 per cent of the hospitalizations, and 27.6 per cent of these were attributed to negligence. In the more recent Australian study, the Quality in Australian Health Care Study (QAHCS; Wilson *et al.*, 1995), a review of the medical records of over 14 000 admissions to 28 hospitals in New South Wales and South Australia revealed that 16.6 per cent of these admissions were associated with an 'adverse event' caused by healthcare management and resulting in disability or a longer stay in hospital. In 1999 a pilot study was carried out in England and, whilst the final analysis is still awaited, early indications suggest a similar incidence to the previous studies. What does this mean in practical terms? In the report of an expert group on learning from adverse events, set up by the Chief Medical Officer and published in June 2000 (DoH, 2000), the figure for adverse events in the United Kingdom in which harm is caused to patients was estimated at a rate of in excess of 850 000 a year or 10 per cent of hospital admissions, costing the NHS £2 billion a year in additional hospital stays alone. The report also goes on to confirm that the NHS has not been good at learning from its mistakes, and that this must be one of the goals for the future.

Health professionals have been placed in an unenviable position because of this failure to acknowledge that adverse events represent a very significant problem in healthcare provision. The response has been one of blame rather than tackling the underlying causes. This is highlighted not least by the fact that to date no central statistics have been kept in the United Kingdom on adverse events, and recording at local level is at best patchy. Until more recently, the main driving force for instituting risk management within the health service has not been patient focused so much as litigation focused. It was only after the setting up of the National Health Service Litigation Authority that risk management first began to be taken seriously, and it still represents more of a fire fighting exercise than a systematic approach to changing practices across the NHS. The only statistics that were available and visible were those arising out of the small proportion of damaged patients who had the wherewithal to seek redress through the courts. Unfortunately, with the focus on litigation a disturbing distortion took place whereby the health service was seen as the victim of litigious patients. This not only ignored the fact that the numbers that litigated represented merely a small proportion of the overall numbers of medical accident victims; it also deflected attention away from the real issue, which was the frequency with which avoidable adverse events were taking place. The focus was primarily on reducing the resulting litigation, far less on failures in care that gave rise to litigation. It also ignored the hidden costs associated with medical accidents, which have only now been acknowledged and recognized as being likely to be far more significant than those associated with litigation.

It is becoming more generally accepted that to concentrate solely on the actions of the health professional who was ultimately responsible for the adverse event is not going to solve the problem or prevent a repetition of the same mistake by a colleague. This is not to say that individuals should not be held accountable where appropriate, but a more effective approach is to analyse what allowed that health professional to make the error and identify what changes are required to minimize the risks of a similar mistake being made in the future. This approach allows for more openness and rather than being punitive, which has tended to be the case, becomes a constructive learning process.

When we look more specifically at obstetric care, this is one of the few areas where there has been some attempt to record and analyse adverse events in the form of the *Confidential Enquiry into Stillbirths and Death in Infancy* (CESDI) and the *Confidential Enquiry into Maternal Deaths*. These make for uncomfortable reading. In the 6th Annual Report published by CESDI in June 1999 (MCHRC, 1999), the average mortality rate by region for stillbirths and deaths during the neonatal and post-neonatal period was 11.3 per 1000 total births (live births totalled at 666 370). In reviewing cases, the CESDI has established an overall grading system for sub-optimal care:

0   No sub-optimal care
1   Sub-optimal care, but different management would have made no
     difference to the outcome
2   Sub-optimal care, but different management might have made a
     difference to the outcome
3   Sub-optimal care where different management would reasonably have
     been expected to have made a difference to the outcome.

In the 1996–1997 review published in the 6th Annual Report, a sample group was selected according to the following criteria: 1 kg or over, 24 weeks' gestation or over, no known congenital abnormalities, and 27 days old or less at the time of death. Of the 5930 notifications in this group, a 1 in 10 random sample was taken ('the sample') to give a final figure of 573 (422 stillbirths and 151 neonatal deaths) cases for a detailed review.

With respect to the stillbirths in the sample, 81 per cent were classified as 'unexplained'. However, 45 per cent of the unexplained group were given a sub-optimal care grade of 2 or 3, and this suggests that 'unexplained' does not necessarily equate to 'unavoidable'. Intrapartum deaths (15 per cent of the sample) provide even more disturbing statistics: 73 per cent of such deaths were graded 2 or 3. What does this mean in real terms? In 22 per cent of the sample (124 cases out of 573) an overall grade of 3 was given, which would suggest that the standard of care was implicated as a causative factor in the outcome of the pregnancy. If this is extrapolated to the full sample group it indicates over 1200 potentially avoidable stillbirths and neonatal deaths a year, and this in itself is likely to prove a conservative estimate. This does perhaps put into perspective the implication that the problem in obstetric care is one of parental expectation.

Clearly there remain some worrying statistics that do not take account of all the 'near misses' – the babies who suffer hypoxic brain damage and other forms of injury at birth. On this basis, it must be recognized that, as with other areas of health care, there is little cause for complacency with respect to the standards operating within the maternity services and that there are a significant number of parents who have genuine grounds for complaint. This should not be interpreted simply as a censure on those who work within the professions, as it is clear that the problems go much deeper.

The role of Action for Victims of Medical Accidents in advising parents

Obstetric cases represent the largest group of enquiries that Action for Victims of Medical Accidents (AVMA) deals with through its advisory service. Parents are usually able to provide sufficiently accurate histories from which it is possible to make a reasonable assessment of the nature of any adverse event and the immediate causative factors. This can be confirmed subsequently by a review of the records and, in those cases that proceed to a legal investigation, by the opinions provided by medical experts instructed to report on the standard of care.

AVMA deals with enquiries involving all aspects of obstetric care, but a significant number relate to stillbirths and cases of cerebral palsy. Other signifi-cant areas include Erb's palsy and injuries to the mother – both psychological and physical. For the families involved, what should have been the happiest event in their lives can prove to be deeply traumatic, entailing long-lasting consequences for the whole family.

Reviewing obstetric cases

In reviewing obstetric cases, the underlying causative factors often follow a familiar pattern. Near the top of the list are professionals working outside their competency, whether this be midwives failing to recognize the need to defer to a more experienced colleague or clinician, or a junior doctor making decisions that are clearly outside his or her training or experience. Protocols, whilst an essential tool, can become dangerous if followed blindly or without the intervention of common sense. There are a significant number of cases where the record keeping is of a good standard and monitoring is carried out in accordance with recommended practice, but there is a complete failure to act on the information that is being recorded.

Case study A: Mrs C

Mrs C was an 'elderly primigravida'. She had a history of infertility, but eventually, following IVF treatment, found that she was pregnant. This was a precious and much-wanted baby.

The pregnancy was uneventful and Mrs C was admitted, in labour, at term. The fetal head was not engaged and labour was slow and prolonged. The labour was augmented with syntocinon. At full dilatation the head was at the level of the ischial spines and remained there.

Mrs C asked for a Caesarean section a number of times, but the midwives did not call the obstetrician. Two further vaginal examinations were performed before the obstetrician was called. By this time Mrs C had been in the second stage for 6 hours. An attempt was made to deliver the baby by forceps, but an emergency Caesarean section was performed where a stillborn boy was delivered.

Mrs C is unable to have any more children.

Mrs C complained to the Trust, with the assistance of the Community Health Council, about her treatment by the midwives. The Trust instigated an investigation, and as a result a number of midwives were disciplined. Mrs C found the Trust to be open and honest with her, admitting that mistakes were made and putting in place procedures to minimize the risk of this occurring again.

The use of oxytocics, particularly in relation to induction of labour, is frequently implicated in hypoxic injury to the fetus resulting in death or serious brain injury. In the presence of a previous Caesarean scar, the particular risks of induction often appear to be overlooked even when the early warning signs of rupture and/or hyperstimulation develop (see case study B).

Case study B: Mrs D

Mrs D was pregnant with her second child. Her first child had been delivered by Caesarean section, but it was thought that this was for a non-recurring reason.

It was recognized throughout her antenatal care that, in addition to the scar on her uterus, she had a number of risk factors, and that she would require careful monitoring during labour. However, no plan was recorded as to the level of monitoring required, how long she was to be allowed to labour, or the use of oxytocics.

She was admitted in labour at term. The midwife was not aware of the previous Caesarean section. Progress was slow, and syntocinon was ordered by the SHO, over the telephone. He was not informed of the uterine scar. The fetal heart rate was recorded at intermittent intervals; there was no continuous recording.

After 10 hours in labour Mrs D began to experience continuous low abdominal pain. The membranes ruptured spontaneously and the liquor was bloodstained. The syntocinon was not decreased but instead increased as per the unit protocol. There was a changeover of midwife at this time, but the new midwife was not informed of the previous Caesarean section. There was a gap of 45 minutes during which there were no recordings of any observations of either fetal or maternal wellbeing.

There was a sudden gush of heavily bloodstained liquor, and Mrs D cried out with severe continuous abdominal pain. The fetal heart was recorded at 50 bpm. The syntocinon was stopped and the registrar called as a matter of urgency.

When it was recognized that there was scar dehiscence an emergency Caesarean section was performed, where the fetus was found to be in the abdominal cavity. Mrs D's uterus had ruptured to such an extent that a hysterectomy had to be performed.

The baby was resuscitated and transferred to SCBU, where she was ventilated. She suffered a cardiac arrest and died 5 days later.

Mrs D's recovery was slow. She was profoundly shocked not only at the loss of her beautiful baby daughter but also by the awful realization that the hysterectomy had removed any chance she may have had of having another baby. Her grief was such that she was not able to speak about her experiences for over a year.

Mrs D could not return to the Trust for follow-up care, and all further care was provided by her GP and the community midwives. The consultant from the Trust tried to contact Mrs D on a number of occasions, both in writing and on the telephone, but Mrs D felt unable to respond. She did not initiate a formal complaint, nor did she instruct solicitors. A number of years later Mrs D felt strong enough to write to the Trust asking for an explanation as to what had happened to her and her baby.

Although Mrs D was well outside the time limit for bringing a complaint under the NHS Complaints Procedure, the Trust did not hesitate to respond to her request for a meeting. The consultant and senior midwife met with Mrs D at her home, at Mrs D's request, and discussed with her the events of her labour and delivery. The Trust recognized and apologized for its failings, particularly in relation to communication between the different health carers. Mrs D had been let down very badly by those caring for her during the antenatal period and her labour and delivery. Not only had there been a failure to communicate, but also no one person had taken overall control and recognized that Mrs D was a high-risk patient. As a result the Trust had acted immediately to put in place procedures and protocols in the labour room to increase awareness and try and reduce the chances of a recurrence of this failure. Mrs D was given a copy of the new protocols.

It is surprising and very worrying that the interpretation or, more accurately, the misinterpretation of CTG traces continues to be one of the commonest factors in avoidable injury or death to the baby. This has been regularly highlighted in the CESDI reports. This raises a number of questions, not least regarding the quality of training in this field for midwives and junior doctors, given the extensive use of electronic monitoring and the false sense of security that it can impart. The question might also be raised as to why the technology is not in place to minimize the risks of human error in the interpretation of the trace.

Locum doctors in obstetrics are a particular cause for concern, as their experience and competency is often untested. There have been some very disturbing cases where the standard of care was such that it could lead to questioning whether the individuals concerned had any appreciable obstetric experience.

Underlying many cases is the failure to listen to the parents (see case studies C and D). A great deal is said about communication within the health service, and in particular between health professionals and patients. However, this often appears to be thought of as giving information and obtaining the woman's consent. Far less emphasis appears to be placed on actively listening to her and in turn using this information to inform clinical decision making.

Case study C: Ms E

Ms E had a normal vaginal delivery. Prior to leaving the unit she was seen and examined independently by two midwives who pronounced her fit for discharge.

Over the next few days at home she was visited by the community midwife. Ms E informed the midwife that she felt 'something was hanging out', and the midwife examined her perineum and pushed whatever it was back into her vagina. The next day a different midwife saw her and Ms E told her of difficulty in passing urine and in walking. She was told to concentrate on doing her pelvic floor exercises.

She started to notice that she had an offensive discharge, and began to take several baths a day because she was so self-conscious about the smell. She became unwell with a high temperature and contacted her GP, who referred her to the A&E department at her local hospital.

Subsequently it was found that she had a retained vaginal swab, and she was given a course of antibiotics.

Ms E was so shocked by what had happened to her and the distressing symptoms she had had to endure that she immediately made a complaint to the Trust. The Trust responded with a standard letter, which did little to satisfy her that a full investigation had been carried out. Ms E requested a meeting with the head of midwifery. At this meeting, Ms E found her attitude to be defensive and wholly supportive of the care provided by the midwives. Ms E became more and more frustrated with the whole process and eventually gave up. She never received an apology or an acknowledgement of the suffering and distress she had experienced.

The impact of a medical accident

The impact of a medical accident on an individual can be significant, particularly where this is not recognized by the health professionals caring for them. The nature of the relationship between patients and health providers is one founded on trust, where the individual places his or her life and wellbeing into the hands of another. If something then goes wrong, particularly where it is evident that not everything was done that should have been, that breach of trust can have a profound impact on the patient and their relatives. In becoming a patient, control is handed over to someone else; when that act of trust is perceived to have been broken or abused, the feelings of powerlessness and loss of control can be both incapacitating and deeply damaging to the patient's self-esteem and confidence. A significant part of recovering from such an event is about regaining control. This can take different forms, but can only really begin when the patient has some understanding of what has happened.

In the aftermath of an adverse outcome occurring during pregnancy or childbirth, in addition to providing support to help the parents cope with the trauma, one of the most important issues from the parents' perspective is information regarding what happened and why. Being told that their baby suffered a lack of oxygen and did not survive labour is not enough. They need to understand why their baby did not survive, what could have been done, and what should have been done. If the outcome was caused by a failure in the delivery of care, they need this to be openly investigated and acknowledged. It is wrong to assume that parents are not aware when mistakes have been made, and if it is seen that healthcare providers are trying to hide information from them, this will only serve to compound the breach of trust.

An apology is an important part of acknowledging what has happened, but this will be perceived as empty if nothing is then done to correct the mistakes that were made. Parents need to know that their loss is being taken sufficiently seriously to lead to corrective action being taken. This is very important. Where no discernible action is taken, this is interpreted as meaning that what happened to them is being dismissed as being of no consequence. Consider any major incident, such as the Clapham rail crash, or the sinking of the *Marchioness* on the Thames. People who have been involved in a traumatic event or loss need the circumstances to be fully investigated and to have any failings acknowledged in order to make some sort of sense of what has happened to them and therefore to begin coming to terms with it. No amount of counselling will replace the deep-seated need to understand what happened. Unfortunately, this generally appears not to be appreciated in the context of health care, despite the fact that many such patients are left deeply traumatized by their experiences.

This is particularly true in the context of obstetric care because, unlike most other areas of health care, the outcome is usually not expected to be anything other than a normal happy event. To be faced with the trauma of an intrapartum stillbirth or a baby suffering the consequences of hypoxia can be the trigger for significant psychological and emotional sequelae. This also applies to what might be considered as 'near misses'. There is often a failure to appreciate that even where both the mother and baby are well, if the delivery has been traumatic and the mother has experienced feelings of loss of control and has feared for her life or that of her baby, she (and her partner) may well be traumatized (see case study D).

Case study D: Mrs A

Mrs A was pregnant with her first child. She was 150 cm (4 ft 11 in) tall, and was told by the midwife at the booking clinic that she would probably require a Caesarean section. However, at further clinic appointments, when seen and examined by both the obstetricians and the midwives, Mrs A was told repeatedly that a Caesarean section would not be necessary. Although she expressed her fears as to her own health and that of her unborn child, these fears were dismissed as being unfounded.

At term the head was floating 'high and free' above the brim of the pelvis, and numerous comments were made in the notes regarding this being a large baby. No plans were made as to a trial of labour, and again Mrs A's fears were dismissed. She found the midwives to be unsympathetic. She was allowed to go past term, and was admitted at 42 weeks for induction of labour.

On admission, a note was again made that this appeared to be a large baby and on palpation the head was high above the brim of the pelvis. Prostaglandin induction was attempted six times but failed. Mrs A was becoming more and more distressed at the number of vaginal examinations that were being performed. She again requested a Caesarean section, but was told how dangerous this would be for the baby and that she was being selfish. Although it was outside their own protocol, a further three attempts at induction were made before a decision was made to perform a Caesarean section. The attempted inductions had taken place over a period of 3 days, during which time more than 15 vaginal examinations were performed. Mrs A found the midwives difficult to talk to and unsupportive.

The baby was delivered in good condition, but Mrs A was profoundly affected by the whole experience and has gone on to develop a significant psychiatric illness.

It took a number of months before Mrs A was able to talk about her experience, and she did not feel able to complain to the hospital involved. The thought of having to return to the hospital for a meeting filled her with dread and she preferred to put the whole matter into the hands of a solicitor, who would be able to put some distance between her and the Trust. However, she found the litigation experience extremely stressful, having to go over and over the trauma of the labour, and could not continue with it. She is still receiving counselling.

Stillbirths

Intrapartum stillbirths are a particular instance where health professionals need to be proactive in their approach to responding to the needs of the parents. The Stillbirth and Neonatal Death Society (SANDS) has produced very helpful guidelines for health professionals in supporting parents after a baby has died (Kohner, 1995). However, an essential part of that support should also include responding to the particular needs of parents where an adverse event may have played a part in the loss of their baby. In this situation, a proactive approach to responding to the parents' concerns is an essential part of the support process. In too many cases, parents are left bewildered by the lack of an acknowledgement or explanation, and health professionals uncomfortable in the knowledge that information is being withheld and that the underlying problems in their maternity services remain unresolved. Case study E is an illustration of the damage that results from not acknowledging mistakes and from withholding information.

Case study E: Mrs G

Mrs G, a 38-year-old woman, arrived at the maternity unit at 9.30 am, having previously telephoned with a history of ruptured membranes. This was her second pregnancy after a gap of 17 years. It was an hour before she was assessed and subsequently placed on a monitor. The midwife in charge of her care was reported to have been sitting across the room reading items out of the newspaper to the patient. The patient, who had a very detailed memory of events, could not recall any review of the CTG trace. At 12.30 am, the registrar happened to be passing the room and took a glance at the CTG record. She identified severe fetal distress with a baseline fetal heart rate of 60 beats per minute. The mother then experienced the trauma of knowing that her baby was in danger, and the alarm of an emergency Caesarean section where there was no pre-warning. A stillborn infant was delivered just after 1.00 pm. Mrs G received conflicting information regarding whether her baby was stillborn or in fact had lived for a short time. She then developed a severe wound infection and remained in hospital for an additional 3 weeks. The staff provided the normal support following a stillbirth, but no one came to explain what had happened. Mrs G subsequently described how she left the hospital unaccompanied, feeling totally isolated and without having any understanding of why she was not leaving with her baby.

The consultant saw Mrs G at her postnatal appointment. Mrs G tried to ask questions, but the consultant responded by quoting stillbirth statistics and reassured her that her case fell into the majority of cases that were unexplained. From her own recollection of events she was not prepared to accept this explanation, and with the assistance of the Community Health Council made a formal complaint in writing. In the hospital's final response 18 months later, they went as far as admitting that there were some changes on the CTG trace but even if this had been recognized earlier, it would have made no difference. In desperation, Mrs G then sought the advice of a solicitor. Her mental state had clearly deteriorated by this stage and included a belief, which arose from the conflicting information over whether her baby was stillborn or not, that something untoward happened or was done to her baby after delivery. She was experiencing flashbacks and also revealed that at night the only place she felt safe and where she could escape from the nightmares was under the stairs.

A preliminary expert's report from a consultant obstetrician identified that had the CTG been reviewed earlier, it was more probable than not that the baby would have been delivered undamaged. Four years after the loss of her baby, her claim for clinical negligence was finally settled. This was of little comfort to the mother, who by this stage had developed a morbid grief reaction and continued to suffer quite severe symptoms of post-traumatic stress disorder. It was not until the case had concluded that the mother could contemplate visiting her baby's grave because of the guilt she felt at not protecting her child and because the issues surrounding his death were unresolved.

It is perhaps self-evident that a more proactive approach would have resulted in a better outcome for all concerned. As it was, the mother and the staff concerned were all embroiled in a lengthy investigation, both through the complaints procedure and litigation, and Mrs G was left with longstanding psychiatric problems. Mrs G was a patient, and her needs after the events in question were as great if not greater than her needs before. Unfortunately, this was not recognized or addressed by any of those involved in her care.

The impact of a lengthy investigation, particularly in relation to stillbirths, means that the grieving process goes on hold, and it is only at its conclusion that the process begins of coming to terms with what has happened. It could be argued that it would be better if people were dissuaded from pursuing such an investigation, but this is not the answer either because they still need to understand what happened. An example of this is a woman who sought advice in relation to an intrapartum stillbirth that had taken place 20 years previously. Following the loss of her baby, she had gone repeatedly to try and speak to the consultant but without success. Eventually she gave up, but developed severe depression that kept her more or less housebound over the next 19 years. The lady subsequently had to go for gynaecological treatment, having put it off for many years. The consultant realized that she had more deep-seated problems, and this eventually led to him accessing her old obstetric records. He very carefully went through these with her and explained what had happened and why her baby had died. This was the first step in enabling her to come to terms with her loss.

Investigation of complaints

So what are the options for parents who have concerns about their care during pregnancy or delivery? The first would be to make a complaint using the NHS Complaints Procedure introduced in 1996. This is a two-stage procedure, comprising a local resolution stage where the complaint is dealt with internally, and an Independent Review where the complaint is subject to review by a panel. Under local resolution patients should be able to raise concerns with any member of staff, who should either deal with it on the spot or refer it to an appropriate person – in many instances the Trust's complaints manager – for investigation. An important source of advice for patients at this stage is their local Community Health Council, or AVMA, where the issues are of a clinical nature.

One of the flaws in local resolution is that often the person dealing with the complaint has no clinical knowledge, limited training in carrying out a clinical investigation, and insufficient status or support within the organization to enable him or her to carry out the sort of detailed investigation required. This has begun to change, but there is still a long way to go. It is therefore not surprising that patients are frequently left dissatisfied with the investigation and the outcome of their complaint. Certainly one obvious answer in relation to clinical complaints would be for healthcare providers to seek an independent clinical opinion at an early stage. This has a number of benefits, not least in acting as a form of external audit.

If patients are dissatisfied with the response to their complaint under local resolution, they can request an independent review. There is no automatic right to an independent review, the decision being made by a convenor – a non-executive director of the Trust or health authority. If the convenor agrees to an independent review, in the case of clinical complaints two independent clinical assessors will be appointed to advise the review panel. Independent reviews can be beneficial, but have been subject to a great deal of criticism. The final arbiter overseeing the functioning of the NHS procedure is the Health Service Ombudsman, who can intervene once local procedures have been exhausted.

A report published by the Public Law Project (Wallace *et al.*, 1999), following research into the NHS complaints procedure, identified many significant failings in the operation of the procedure and made a number of recommendations. There are changes that, if implemented, could well improve the functioning of the procedure, but what is essential is a change in the attitude to responding to complaints and, more particularly, adverse clinical events. In theory there is no reason why the present procedure should not work satisfactorily if minimizing the risks of adverse events is recognized as fundamental to the delivery of safe health care, and the needs of patients in this situation are recognized and dealt with as a priority.

Case history F: Mrs E

Mrs E's labour and delivery were conducted solely by midwives. An episiotomy was performed and sutured by the midwife.

Immediately post-delivery, Mrs E experienced problems with passing flatus and urgency when defaecating. She did not tell the midwives, believing that these problems were due to the delivery and would settle down in time.

After being discharged home Mrs E was cared for by the community midwives. She was visited each day and regular postnatal observations were made, including examination of the perineum. Concern was expressed by the midwife as to the condition of the perineum, and Mrs E admitted that she had been having problems since delivery. These had had such an effect on her that she was finding it difficult bonding with her new baby and was afraid to leave the house because of soiling herself in public. The midwife called in the GP, who immediately referred Mrs E back to hospital.

Mrs E required surgery to repair the external anal sphincter, and for formation of a temporary colostomy. It was a year before this was reversed, but she is not fully continent and will need a Caesarean section for future deliveries. She has also suffered psychological injury as a result of the midwife failing to recognize the third degree tear, and continues to require counselling.

Mrs E's family encouraged her to complain and, with the help of her local Community Health Council, she lodged a complaint. Unfortunately this was well outside the 6-month time limit for bringing a complaint under the NHS Complaints procedure, and the Trust refused to investigate. Mrs E complained to the Health Service Ombudsman, who was also loath to interfere. Eventually, after pressure from various quarters, the Trust carried out a limited investigation that supported the midwife's actions. Mrs E requested a meeting, but this was refused and Mrs E felt she had no alternative but to report the midwife to the UKCC. She found the whole experience extremely stressful, and after some time felt that she did not have the energy to take her complaint any further.

Private patients

Private patients who have been treated in an independent hospital face even more of a problem when it comes to making a complaint. The NHS Complaints Procedure does not apply unless the patient is an NHS patient being treated in the independent sector or in a private bed in an NHS Trust. Most large private hospitals should abide by the Independent Healthcare Associations' recently published code of practice for handling complaints (IHA, 2000). One of the main flaws in the investigation of private complaints is that it is difficult to achieve a comprehensive investigation because the patient's consultant is normally an independent contractor. Until very recently, patients were expected to complain directly to their treating consultant. With the introduction of clinical governance, independent hospitals should now be expected to accept responsibility for their admitting consultants, which in theory should include the investigation of all aspects of a clinical complaint. The Health Service Ombudsman has no jurisdiction where private patients are unhappy with the outcome of their complaint, but patients can request an investigation by the local health authority although their powers are currently very limited. New legislation for the regulation of the independent sector is expected imminently.

A proactive response to adverse clinical events

There is a strong argument to suggest that the complaints procedures should have very little part to play when it comes to the investigation of an adverse event. It clearly has a place in more minor complaints, or the sort of complaints where the staff would not necessarily be in a position to identify that there was a problem. However, with respect to adverse clinical events, the present situation is such that patients are generally unlikely to get a full explanation unless they have the wherewithal to pursue a formal complaint.

In the context of obstetric care and a significant adverse event, if practitioners sit back and wait for people to complain, that initial silence has two significant consequences. First, it greatly compounds the trauma and distress that the parents experience and makes it very difficult for them to come to terms with what has happened. It may also appear to them that the absence of an open inquiry process is indicative that what has happened is not being treated with the gravity it deserves. This can be deeply hurtful and potentially damaging because it increases their sense of powerlessness. Secondly, by remaining silent or offering only a partial explanation, practitioners may lose the patient's trust. The silence may well be interpreted, rightly or wrongly, as a 'cover-up'. The consequences of this are that should an explanation be offered some weeks or months later, the patient is going to find it difficult to accept in the light of the initial silence.

AVMA has for many years advocated a proactive approach to responding to adverse events. This means that instead of waiting to see whether the patient complains, as soon as an adverse event is identified an immediate investigation that includes the patient and/or relatives is instituted. Such an approach has been tried in the USA. In the Veterans' Affairs Medical Centre in Lexington, after two substantial law suits were lost, a proactive policy was introduced to ensure the early identification and investigation of accidents and incidents of medical negligence (Kraman and Hamm, 1999). Having introduced this policy, an ethical issue arose when incidents were identified of which the patient or next of kin was unaware. The risk management committee decided that in such cases the facility had a duty to remain in the 'role of caregiver' and should notify the patient of the committee's findings. The initial findings suggest that adopting this form of 'honest and forthright' approach, which is referred to as a 'humanistic' risk management policy, has a number of benefits, not least (but perhaps most surprisingly) reducing litigation costs.

If health providers do adopt a proactive approach to identifying and investigating adverse events, the investigation should move away from simply targeting individual health professionals. Whilst individuals may ultimately be culpable, there are sufficient data to suggest that attention needs to be focused on the systems within which those health professionals work and the sort of failures in those systems that lead to human error (Bogner, 1994). Such failures may include, for example, systems that allow people to make decisions beyond their competency or experience, unsafe staffing levels, poor resourcing resulting in faulty or substandard equipment, poor communication between health professionals, inadequate protocols, people working when they are overtired or stressed etc. An investigation sufficiently rigorous to identify such failures is not an easy task, and requires people trained to carry out such investigations, but is essential if the underlying causes are to be addressed. The present reality is that the true causes of an adverse event often remain undisclosed. Individual healthcare professionals may well be disciplined, but this will not in itself prevent one of their colleagues from making the same mistake.

Clinical negligence litigation

Pursuing a legal claim for clinical negligence should ideally be the option of last resort, but for many patients it is perceived as the only option. The reasons for this are complex. It is generally accepted that society has in general become more ready to resort to the law in order to resolve disputes. Solicitors have largely shaken off their unapproachable image with high street shop fronts and widespread advertising. Meanwhile the increasing number of consumer programmes reiterate and reinforce the compensation message. Patients who have been injured often feel that they are powerless against the institutions that harmed them, particularly if there has been a failure to acknowledge the harm that has been done. Many do not have the reserves or stamina to fight their way through the complaints procedures, and often have little faith in the outcome. A dismissive response or inadequate explanation will drive patients to seek recompense, and the most obvious recourse is through the power of the law.

For a significant number of patients, compensation is seen as a necessity – to provide for a child who will never lead an independent life or to compensate for the loss of a parent and the care that they would have provided. For others, it represents a more tangible form of acknowledgement for what has happened to them. For the latter group the money itself is often of little import, but what it represents is significant. The fact that some patients will push for the maximum damages is often interpreted as meaning that money is the ultimate goal. However, the compensation is often not so much about the original incident but rather about the way in which they were treated after the event. Compensation comes to represent all the things that they believed should have happened as a matter of course after the accident – the investigation, the acknowledgement, the apology, and the reassurance that the same mistake would not be repeated.

For healthcare professionals, medical litigation is largely perceived as a threat. This is understandable, particularly where a culture of blame exists – arising not so much from patients as from within the health service itself. As discussed earlier, this sort of fear and misconception stems from the failure within our health services to address adverse events in a pragmatic and systematic way. People would not normally question the rights of a pedestrian to receive compensation for being made paraplegic as a result of a momentary lapse in attention of a car driver. These sorts of accidents happen, and we make contingencies for them. The attitude is generally very different when it comes to those injured during the course of medical treatment. The nature of health care does mean that an adverse outcome can be wrongly interpreted by patients as a negligent outcome. If, for example, there is a catalogue of errors during the delivery of a baby and that baby is subsequently found to have cerebral palsy, then it is understandable that the mother might believe there is a causal connection – particularly if the problems during the delivery were not addressed at the time. This goes back to the point that much could be done to alleviate the burden of litigation, not least by introducing effective systems for the early identification and investigation of adverse events.

Legal action is by no means the easy option for patients, particularly where they have suffered a traumatic event. The process requires the individual concerned to revisit the events in question, to have every detail of their medical history scrutinized, and, at its conclusion, to come to terms with the realization that financial compensation is not going to turn the clock back and take away the loss that has been suffered. Patients also face all the uncertainties that litigation can present. Establishing that the standard of care was negligent – i.e. was below the standard of practice normally expected of a practitioner in that field – is only half the battle. It then has to be established that the act or acts of negligence were directly responsible for the injuries suffered. This is referred to as causation. This is very much to the forefront with respect to claims involving hypoxia at birth and the development of cerebral palsy. For a claim to succeed, it has to be established, on the balance of probabilities, that the damage could have been avoided but for the negligence in care. There are many cases where it is difficult to prove this causal link because of arguments such as the injury having existed before the event in question, or because it cannot be proved that different treatment would have prevented the injury taking place – for example, in the case of placental abruption.

The new Civil Procedure Rules and the Pre-action Protocol

The introduction of the new Civil Procedure Rules in April 1999 was a positive step forward for both patients and the health service. These rules govern the conduct of civil claims including claims for clinical negligence. The main thrust of the new rules is to achieve early settlement of claims, and to avoid unnecessary litigation wherever possible.

An important part of this was the introduction of a clinical negligence pre-action protocol. The protocol sets out guidelines for best practice during the preliminary stages of investigating a claim for clinical negligence before court proceedings have been commenced. It encourages a climate of openness when something has 'gone wrong' with a patient's treatment, as well as recommending a timed sequence of steps for patients and healthcare providers to follow when a dispute arises. It doesn't just deal with procedural issues, but also tries to encourage an alternative approach to dealing with potential claims.

Under the protocol healthcare providers are expected to ensure that they have clinical governance strategies in place, including the early identification and investigation of adverse events. They should advise patients of a serious adverse outcome and provide, on request, a written or oral explanation of what happened. Patients in turn should report any concerns to the healthcare provider as soon as is reasonable and should consider the full range of options open to them in addition to litigation. If, having investigated the matter, the patient/adviser decides that there are grounds for a claim, he or she must send a 'letter of claim' to the health provider/potential defendant detailing the allegations and the injuries and losses suffered by the patient. This then gives the defendant an opportunity to investigate and, if appropriate, settle the claim before both parties become involved in expensive legal proceedings. Both parties have the option of putting forward an offer to settle at this stage. If the parties are unable to reach agreement under the pre-action protocol and the patient/adviser is satisfied that there are grounds for a claim, the next step is then to issue legal proceedings.

As can be seen, this is very much in line with the proactive approach discussed above. There is already some anecdotal evidence to suggest that an increasing number of claims are being settled prior to legal proceedings, reducing much of the burden faced by health professionals and patients, both financial and emotional. It also recognizes the duty owed to patients who have been injured, and avoids much of the adversarial approach that has dominated the legal system in the past.

The future

We are now entering a new era where, it is hoped, minimizing the risks of adverse events will be at the top of the healthcare agenda. It should not only inform all policy initiatives; it should be the bedrock of healthcare provision. By introducing a systematic approach to collecting and analysing data, it should then be possible to begin tackling both the causes and the consequences of adverse events. This includes both the impact on health professionals as well as the trauma and injury experienced by the patients involved who look to those health professionals to provide the answers. Without this approach, patients will continue to become victims twice over – both of the error and of the failure to address their needs afterwards.

Where error is identified and admitted, it is important to accept that patients are entitled to claim compensation. It is a big step to move from the present defensiveness to a situation where error can be openly acknowledged and the rights of patients who have been harmed met. However, the seeds of change have already been sown, and the future looks more promising both for patients and their health carers who carry an unnecessarily heavy burden for the failures in our health services.

References

Bogner, M. S. (ed.). (1994). *Human Error in Medicine*. Lawrence Erlbaum Associates.

Brennan, T. A., Leape, L. L., Laird, N. *et al.* (1991). Incidence of adverse events and negligence in hospitalised patients: results of the Harvard Medical Practice Study I. *N. Engl. J. Med.*, **324**, 370–76.

Department of Health (2000). *An Organization with a Memory*. HMSO.

Independent Healthcare Association (2000). *Handling Patients' Complaints: A Code of Practice for Members of the IHA*. IHA.

Kohner, N. (1995). *Pregnancy, Loss and the Death of a Baby: Guidelines for Professionals*. SANDS.

Kraman, S. S. and Hamm, G. (1999). Risk management: extreme honesty may be the best policy. *Ann. Int. Med.*, **131(12)**, 963–7.

Maternal and Child Health Research Consortium (1999). *Confidential Enquiry into Stillbirth and Death in Infancy*, 6th Report. MCHRC.

Wallace, H., Mulcahy, L. and Ashton, K. (1999). *The NHS Complaints Procedure 3 Years On: An Evaluation of the Operation and Effectiveness of Complaints Management in the NHS*. Public Law Project.

Wilson, R. McL., Runciman, W. B., Gibberd, R. W. *et al.* (1995). The Quality in Australian Health Care Study. *Med. J. Aust.*, **163**, 458–71.

11

The way forward: clinical competence, co-operation and communication

Andrew Symon and Jo Wilson

Introduction

This final chapter summarizes some of the points made in this book, and leads the reader through some of the conclusions that can be drawn from the evidence presented here. The chapter begins by giving an overview of the argument about what clinical risk management is doing, and whether it can guarantee the right to a perfect baby. It then goes on to suggest ways in which the practitioner can help the risk management process, with particular reference to the new 'Three Cs' – competence, co-operation, and communication. While acknowledging that there are no cast-iron guarantees in maternity care (or in life generally), the chapter argues that a genuine focus on these three complementary aspects of care is the best way forward for practitioners who want to achieve the best for the women and babies who receive their care.

Overview

Society's views about risk and its acceptability appear to be changing. In 1988, Ellis commented: 'A vastly inflated concept of medicine's capacity to overcome all the ills of mankind leads quite a number of people to interpret the right to health care as a right to health'. This was echoed by Huntingford (1990, p. 687), who claimed that: 'A well-informed generation has high expectations of their medical attendants'.

A former Chief Medical Officer confirmed this perception (Acheson, 1991). In a speech to midwives, he talked of how awareness of advances in obstetrics had:

> ... fuelled an unrealistic public expectation that a child who receives optimum care during pregnancy and delivery should not be neurologically impaired ... when an impairment is present it is supposed that the cause is to be found in obstetric mismanagement.

These views hold that while the public's knowledge has increased, this increase has been outstripped by the expectation that, whenever difficulties arise, someone somewhere should be able to deal with them. The view that people always expect others to solve their problems is discussed in Bridges' article in *The Times* (28 January, 1999).

Have people really developed the belief that society has the responsibility of sorting out their problems? It can be argued, paradoxically, that an increasingly sceptical public, fed with stories of rail disasters, food scares, child abduction and incompetent practitioners, appears now to have little faith in the integrity or ability of government, of corporate business (or any large organization), or of humanity in general. The belief that those who run the health service can provide a safe, effective and user-friendly organization has been severely dented by a recent series of well-publicized medical disasters. These range from apparent incompetence in paediatric cardiac surgery in Bristol to allegedly arrogant and inept obstetricians/gynaecologists being disciplined by the General Medical Council, and a GP found guilty of mass murder. Television documentaries such as *Why Doctors make Mistakes* and *Doctors on Trial* increase the recognition of error in healthcare decision-making, and indeed of the predisposition of some organizations to make such errors.

Moore (2000, p.4) asserts that:

> *... experts now believe you are more likely to die as a result of something going wrong in a hospital than in a road accident, an air crash or a fire. Under the cloak of silence that covers medical mishaps, such deaths are rarely discussed – and are even covered up and denied.*

Publicity of this type has induced a siege mentality in some quarters: Bogle (2000) claims that at one stage 'media attacks were being stoked up by ministers with an anti-doctor agenda'. Charles Vincent, of the Clinical Risk Unit at University College London, estimates that clinical blunders in the UK may kill 40 000 people a year, making medical error the third most frequent cause of death after cancer and heart disease (Rogers, 1999). Accident prevention is a well-developed area: many resources have been allocated to preventing accidents in children and the elderly, and to the prevention of suicides. However, the current figure of 40 000 people a year dying from adverse healthcare events is four times more than that for all other types of accident. It also appears to be twice the rate (relative to the size of population) as in the USA: at the Health Economist Conference in London in April 2000 it was stated that 98 000 people die each year from adverse healthcare events in the USA.

Obstetric problems are a major cause of claims in clinical practice. Up to 70 per cent of all claims logged with the Clinical Negligence Scheme for Trusts (CNST) relate to obstetrics and gynaecology (Wilson, 1997). The high value of obstetric claims means that they are responsible for a large portion of the CNST's contingent liability. Recent figures estimate that cerebral palsy and brain damage cases account for 80 per cent of the value of outstanding legal claims (NAO, 2001).

This tells us much about the ready availability of information and commentary in contemporary society. In a changing world, people may be caught between the drive for increased personal freedoms represented by a market-driven global economy, and a desire for the perceived security of a paternalist welfare state. Nevertheless, when it comes to health care, and despite recent concerns over the ability of the medical profession to police itself, most people in Britain would seem still to invest their trust in practitioners, whose competence and ability are generally assumed. While this is mostly good news for midwives (and others working in maternity care), it does make ensuring adequate standards and dealing effectively with poor clinical outcomes all the more imperative.

A developing field

How does this affect clinical risk management in midwifery? It means that the process must now be as transparent as possible. The public has access to information from a variety of media, and it can be assumed that there is a belief that the health service is tackling issues of competence.

The field of clinical risk management is certainly moving on. Under the CNST there are specific standards for maternity services, and many English Trusts have met Level 2 and some have met Level 3, which demonstrates fully integrated clinical risk management initiatives. In April 2000, an NHS Trust in Sheffield initiated what it claimed was probably the first Directorate with a specific responsibility for putting risk management into practice. Among other things, this included specifying risk management objectives in each directorate's annual targets.

In June 2000, the Royal College of Obstetricians and Gynaecologists produced its clinical governance advice paper on clinical risk management for practitioners (RCOG, 2000). This stressed the need to move from risk identification (e.g. collecting data on poor outcomes using clinical indicators as discussed in Chapter 2) to risk control – i.e. 'minimizing the risk of subsequent, similar adverse healthcare events' (RCOG, 2000, p. 5). It was noted in Chapters 1 and 5 that, with the advent of the Department of Health's *A First Class Service: Quality in the New NHS* report (DoH, 1997), practitioners now have an explicit responsibility to demonstrate evidence-based care and a legal duty to demonstrate quality of care.

The process of change can be difficult, and change imposed from above is not always welcome. For those who decide and initiate policy changes there is a need to recognize that those who deliver maternity care, and those who use the service, must be involved. In Chapter 5, Stewart noted the need to provide training for those lay people who are brought in to help develop policy. As with the production and updating of protocols and guidelines, a sense of ownership will make new initiatives much easier to implement. In practice this requires greatly improved communication channels, both between practitioners of different grades and disciplines, and between patient and practitioner.

In essence, then, clinical risk management will be driven forward most effectively by a combination of maintaining and improving clinical competence, and by effective communication. Both of these are underpinned by co-operation, which itself requires mutual respect and much closer team working by all those involved in the delivery of care.

Are midwives good communicators?

In Chapter 4, Thompson detailed the need for effective communication and stressed the force of language, noting that it can be a powerful technique for controlling others. Some of this control may be unwitting and even involuntary, but it is very real nonetheless.

Many midwives may pride themselves on being good communicators, although it is comparatively rare to find hospitals providing training in communication skills. It is often assumed that healthcare practitioners are good at communication, as if the socialization process ensures such proficiency. In practice, and as Thomas and Tansley showed in Chapter 10, very often it is the poor quality of communication from health service staff that patients and their families find most distressing. As stated in Chapters 1 and 2, many problems occur due to deficiencies in communication.

The need for good communication starts very early in the clinical risk management process. Ideally, the woman and her family will have pre-conceptual counselling, although it is acknowledged that very often this is not possible. In Chapter 7, McHale noted the times when pre-conceptual counselling is most likely. Without denigrating the desire to minimize the incidence or effects of serious genetic conditions, it is right to acknowledge that there is a debate about whether genetic testing could and should be used to eliminate so-called 'undesirable' characteristics. In theory, the 'right to a perfect baby' could include determining not only its gender and IQ level, but also its eye colour and facial features. Brave New World indeed.

There is an obvious need to take a detailed history when the pregnant woman first presents to the health service. This is essential risk management: although the emphasis is quite rightly on stressing the essential normality of pregnancy, much of the skill of midwifery lies in recognizing when normality is no longer present (and then, of course, dealing appropriately with the new circumstances).

The location for much of this information gathering may be critical. Sometimes a woman is booked in her own home, and it is likely that she will feel comfortable there and will be more relaxed and forthcoming. In the hospital, by contrast, the setting is probably unfamiliar to her, the midwife is more likely to be (or to appear) rushed, and she may even feel intimidated. The quality of information obtained in such circumstances is not likely to be as good. The skill of the midwife is a vital clinical risk management tool at this crucial first meeting.

At this early opportunity the midwife may identify factors that will affect the future management of the pregnancy. The terms 'high risk' and 'low risk', while routinely used, may be misleading. Midwives should always be aware that risk ratings may change – usually from 'low' to 'higher' – and at any stage in the pregnancy. Again, it is worth stressing that whatever plan of management is decided upon at different stages throughout the pregnancy will be based upon negotiation with the woman. Involving her from the earliest opportunity may be one of the most effective risk management tools available to midwives. As Nolan states in Chapter 9, this requires the midwife to be able to give the kind of information that each woman wants. Continuity of care during the antenatal period should help to foster a trusting relationship, and this is a service that independent midwives in particular offer, albeit at a price.

Leaflets are a commonly used medium for imparting information about antenatal screening procedures or other facilities available in the locality. The needs of the local community must be taken into account when producing such material, and this may mean providing leaflets in several languages and offering the services of an interpreter. Written and other materials need to explain matters in sufficient depth without being overwhelming; equally, they need to be straightforward and uncomplicated without being patronizing. The adverse healthcare events and claims histories of independent midwives demonstrate that women are more satisfied if they receive continuity of care and ongoing communication through effective partnerships (Wilson, 1996).

Trust/customer care

If the materials produced by the health service are informative and effective, they will do much to gain the woman's trust. Thomas and Tansley note in Chapter 10 that most patients still place their trust in those who work for the health service. Nothing, of course, will be more effective in gaining trust than the demeanour, approach and evident capability of the practitioner, whether this is the midwife, GP or obstetrician. This may be called the 'customer care' of NHS patients. The term may seem inappropriate in the healthcare setting: despite the best efforts of those keen to see market forces govern the NHS, the health service is not the same sort of organization as a retail store or restaurant. Some practitioners may point out that the NHS is not a profit-making organization, and that many of the NHS' 'customers' have little choice. Nevertheless, the delivery of services is believed to be more 'customer friendly' nowadays (Clyne and Forlenza, 1997), and 'customer care' training has been imported into the NHS (Chaston, 1994). While its use appears to be rather sporadic, valuable lessons can be learned. With an emphasis on providing choice and ensuring valid consent, the midwife must be able to provide information and care in a way that is, if not attractive, then at least palatable.

Many women will attend for antenatal care having already acquired a large amount of information, and midwives will be well aware of the huge availability of material within the general media. Although magazines and television programmes have been accused by some practitioners of raising expectations to unrealistic levels (Symon 2001), midwives have to acknowledge that women will obtain information about pregnancy and childbirth from a variety of sources. That the portrayal of issues is not always to the liking of practitioners goes without saying (*cf.* Henderson *et al.*, 2000). Dealing with the issues raised in articles or programmes requires practitioners to be sensitive and forthright. Open and honest discussions will do much to build up a trusting relationship.

If the pregnant woman and the midwife trust each other, then consent (see Chapter 6) is not likely to be a problem. Difficulties arise when the midwife has not explained things adequately. There is perhaps an increasing danger of this: while there is a drive to reduce the overall number of antenatal visits for each woman, the amount of information that needs to be imparted is growing. Time management skills, like communication skills, may not figure prominently in the midwifery pre-registration curriculum, or in in-service education thereafter. Nevertheless, they are an important part of effective midwifery practice, and therefore of good clinical risk management.

If midwives can ensure that they communicate effectively with each pregnant woman, and can negotiate with her an acceptable and realistic plan of management for her pregnancy, then it will be much easier to deal with any complications that arise. This is of course much harder to accomplish if the woman refuses the advice given by the midwife. In this case it is the midwife's duty to support the mother, even if she personally disagrees with the woman's point of view. Bar the most exceptional cases (i.e. when the woman is not mentally competent), a woman has the right to refuse any treatment or intervention, even if this will result in her death or that of her unborn baby. Such situations are, thankfully, rare. The midwife will only rarely encounter stern opposition to her suggestions if they are sensible and imparted tactfully.

Having established a relationship of trust and confidence, the woman is much less likely to feel that she has been let down by the service when, for whatever reason, her expectations are not met. Maintaining channels of communication is probably the most effective means of minimizing adverse consequences when a clinical outcome is poor, or when the standard of care is believed to have been low. In practical terms, this means being open and honest about what has happened, and offering explanations and, if appropriate, sincere apologies. There is an understandable reluctance on the part of practitioners to say that they are sorry because of the fear that this may be taken as an admission of guilt (Symon, 2001). However, failing to keep the communication channels open with parents in cases where the outcome is believed or known to be poor will almost certainly make them believe that practitioners are hiding the truth. As noted in Chapter 10, sometimes parents believe the only way they will get a truthful answer is if they employ a solicitor. A perception of flippancy has even led directly to the initiation of a lawsuit that would otherwise have been avoided (Symon, 2001). In effect, practitioners are at times believed to be driving people towards litigation – the very opposite of what is intended. It hardly needs to be said that this is very ineffectual risk management.

Are midwives clinically competent?

Ensuring competent standards in practitioners is a *sine qua non* of clinical risk management: without an adequate standard of clinical care, effective communication is worth little. The responsibility for ensuring that practitioners are competent lies with our educational institutions and the health service itself. Students will learn much from working with qualified midwives, and there is a responsibility to ensure that they are provided with effective practical skills.

In both pre- and post-registration education, there is room to improve clinical risk management. This may not be done explicitly, but effective teaching and education will promote this. One method that is gaining in popularity is combined education for practitioners from different disciplines. Whether this applies to students or qualified staff, there is much to be gained from sharing learning opportunities. At the midwifery pre-registration level, sharing lectures and clinical skills sessions with medical students can do much to prevent building of the barriers that have traditionally existed in clinical practice. This message can be reinforced during in-service sessions for qualified staff. Midwives and doctors often need to learn the same skills (e.g. CTG interpretation or perineal repair), and there is little sense in separate teaching.

As the barriers come down between the different disciplines, so the dangers of territoriality are minimized. In Chapter 4, Thompson described some of the dangers of midwives and doctors not communicating effectively.

Practice must be based on current evidence and research. This is now a familiar refrain, but it is worth stressing. Policies, protocols and guidelines (the terms are used interchangeably in some units), which have been developed by a variety of groups and organizations, must be well referenced and reflect local practicalities. While the notion of equality of care demands that there should be a degree of convergence between clinical practice in different units, there also needs to be room for differences in practice. This is sensitive risk management; a protocol that is too deterministic will disallow professional judgement and leave no room for the individual. Since there is no such thing as a standard pregnant woman or a standard labour, it makes little sense to try and ensure that every pregnancy or labour fits a pre-defined plan.

Protocols and guidelines must be seen (and used) as tools and not rules. The protocol or guideline that leaves no room for the individual carries great danger. Practitioners applying such rules would simply be following a script, and not using their judgement, clinical knowledge or intelligence. The dangers of 'cookbook midwifery' are obvious. To get around this, protocols must be developed with input from different sources. Gone are the days when a senior clinician could sit down and write the unit protocol based on his or her own preferred practice. Input from different disciplines, as well as users of the maternity services, is essential; this will help to ensure that there is a clear rationale behind a protocol, and will help to convey a sense of ownership.

Practitioners are encouraged to get involved in the production and updating of protocols and guidelines. Most protocols and guidelines have a 'shelf life': the 'Green top' guidelines produced by the RCOG have a shelf life of 3 years. After this time they must be reviewed and, if necessary, updated. In addition to being based on sound research and evidence, protocols and guidelines must be fully referenced and dated, and the authors acknowledged. Although protocols and guidelines must be reasonably comprehensive, they must be practical. There have been claims that many hospital protocols and guidelines are bulky documents 'composed of excessive amounts of paperwork, with wording which is incomprehensible or ambiguous. Therefore staff avoid reading and using them' (Taylor-Adams and Lyons, 1998). Impractical protocols and guidelines are poor clinical risk management tools.

Variations in the protocols of different units do not necessarily indicate that one is right and another is wrong; they may simply reflect acceptable differences in practice. The same is true for the various lists relating to critical incidents in this book. An item appearing on one list but not on another does not indicate that one unit is overly anxious to detect something, or that another is not being careful enough. It is quite acceptable for different units to have a slightly different emphasis on what it requires of staff, as long as practitioners comply with reasonable (which now means evidence- or research-based) practice.

There is evidence that the use of guidelines and protocols in the USA can demonstrate improvements over time. MMI Companies Inc. have data from the same group of clients reporting the practice of baseline fetal monitoring over 12 years, which have demonstrated that practice can be improved over time (MMI Companies Inc., 1998). These data have been benchmarked and compared using volume, practice and outcome. A representative change in an important practice pattern is shown in Figure 11.1. The incidence of establishing fetal wellbeing through baseline fetal monitoring when women are admitted to maternity units has significantly improved. Change did not occur instantly: it took several years for the practice pattern to become fully modified. It takes at least 2–3 years to change practice and modify behaviour in line with evidence-based practice and research outcomes. However, once achieved, improvements can be sustained.

The importance of guidelines is also demonstrated when examining whether they have been followed when claims or potential claims arise (Figure 11.2).

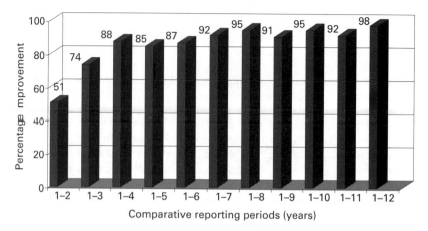

Figure 11.1 Improving practice over time: baseline fetal monitoring (MMI Companies Inc., 1998).

The average cost per claim was 72 times lower when hospitals followed all guidelines ($3002 per claim) compared with when there was no compliance ($218 910) (these losses include indemnity and expenses above and below deductible levels). The pattern remains the same when both open and closed claims are displayed with all reserves and payments included. The middle column demonstrates that when at least some of the guidelines were followed, the average cost per claim was significantly less than when no guidelines are followed.

Protocols and guidelines that are produced by midwives and doctors should also help to break down the barriers between these groups, and promote effective teamwork. Equally, input from users of the service should help to ensure that the point of view of the recipient of care is not forgotten. Stewart notes in Chapter 5 that practice should be based on women's needs as well as current research and evidence. These factors can help to optimize clinical risk management by improving communication and understanding between different people. Just as important, sensitivity shown by practitioners in the clinical setting will help to improve the relationship with the pregnant or labouring woman.

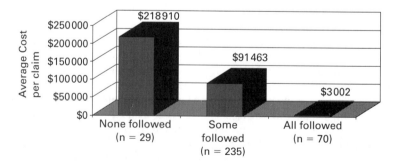

Figure 11.2 Obstetric guideline compliance: closed claims (losses include both indemnity and expense, above and below deductible) (MMI Companies Inc., 1998).

Supervision/reflection

There is a particular difficulty when locum or other short-term staff are employed. Their familiarity with a unit and its protocols, and with the staff there, cannot be taken for granted. Additional supervision for these practitioners is required, whatever their grade.

This brings us on to the need to have adequate supervision for all staff. Midwifery has a long tradition of a formal supervision process, but supervision must extend beyond the formal relationship to encompass peer supervision at all levels. Practitioners from different disciplines can supervise one another.

It should not be necessary to state that the supervision process needs to be positive. While junior practitioners may expect to have a period of mentorship following their registration, it may be harder for more experienced midwives to accept peer supervision. However, being experienced is not necessarily a guarantee of competence, or even of giving adequate care. Cases referred to the UKCC's Professional Conduct Committee sometimes involve very experienced practitioners making very basic errors. These have included poor basic care, rudeness, unnecessary force during examinations, and poor documentation (Anon, 2000). The UKCC is forthright in its assertion that practitioners must report concerns about poor standards in colleagues (UKCC, 1996). Not to do so is a disservice to the women who receive care from that practitioner, and to the practitioner herself, especially if ultimately she faces disciplinary action as a result of her shortcomings.

Reflection is another part of the process of continually reviewing practice. Midwives are encouraged to note what they do, and to reflect on how effective this has been. Questions that can help this process include (see Walters, 2000):

- What was important to me about the last hour on duty?
- Was the particular activity important to me/my client/my colleagues?
- Was I able to influence what was going on? If so, what part did I play? If not, why was this?

These methods aim to ensure that any deficiencies in care are identified and amended. All midwives are human, and can make mistakes. Nobody functions at optimum level all of the time, and there is always room for improvement. Reflection and supervision aim to complement the risk management process by ensuring that the standard of care is under review and that, where necessary, lessons are learnt.

Audit

Audit is another method that can help the clinical risk management process. Whereas reflection is a personal matter, shared (if at all) only with close colleagues, audit is a systematic process that aims to ensure that the standard of care is continually improved. Clinical audit is a crucial tool for ensuring improvements in the quality of patient care. One of the key components of clinical governance (discussed in Chapter 1) is for all clinicians to participate in internal and external clinical audit systems. Clinical audit provides a comprehensive framework for quality improvement activity and processes for monitoring clinical care using effective information and clinical record systems.

An effective clinical audit programme helps to give necessary reassurance to women, clinicians and managers that an agreed quality of service is being provided within available resources. It is performed to improve standards of care, to raise awareness of costs, to eliminate waste and inefficiency, and as a valuable educational tool for peers, juniors and other professionals. It is an educational process for clinicians, identifying inappropriate and inefficient clinical practices and inadequate support. It can lead to increased consumer awareness and choices about health care, as information becomes more readily available about clinical activity, quality of services and health outcomes. Clinical audit has an important role in risk management in revealing where care is ineffective or below acceptable standards, and in encouraging its replacement with effective care and improved clinical outcomes.

Many contracts of employment stipulate the requirement to be involved in critical reviews of clinical care, which in practice often means the audit process. Becoming involved in audit can help midwives to become more aware of their own practice as well as that of their colleagues. Most practitioners have a 'hobby horse' – a view that a particular aspect of care is not done well. This may stem from personal experience – for example, having done things differently in another unit – or from a reading of the research literature. The 'we've always done it this way' culture is under challenge: habits acquired over long periods are not always good habits, and audit is one way of demonstrating that the way in which clinical care is offered can be both different and better.

Professional self-regulation

Clinical audit has an important role in professional self-regulation. It enables clinicians and midwives to hold a mirror to their everyday work and, through discussion with peers and guidance from their professional bodies, make any relevant changes. For this reason the various professional bodies are increasingly requiring that clinical audit is a key component of all specialist training. Health Commissioners and NHS Trusts also need to encourage and support clinicians to include audit in their professional self-regulation and continuing educational development programmes. This involves ensuring that adequate resources (such as protected time and support) are available. It also requires the information and implications of clinical audit studies to be shared. Such information becomes integrated into the clinical risk and clinical governance strategies, and helps to ensure that lessons are learned and shared throughout the healthcare system.

Clinical risk modification

The tools of clinical risk modification, through audit, professional self-regulation, use of clinical guidelines etc., are designed to be proactive and to concentrate on helping the multidisciplinary team to minimize and/or eliminate the cause of potential risk. They should be used to assist professionals in the audit and evaluation of care. If locally owned and controlled, they also serve as a change management mechanism to help maternity units to strive towards the best outcomes.

Members of the multidisciplinary team can begin to apply risk management to their own maternity setting and achieve risk modification in the following ways:

- *Awareness and evaluation.* An in-depth assessment of the maternity services and practices, and costs related to each, can begin to provide data on which potential risk areas can be identified. Included in this identification process are both the clinical and non-clinical components of the organization that contribute to the overall episode of care. Awareness is the first phase of risk modification.
- *Education and implementation.* The development of processes and interventions that begin to change undesirable practices is the second phase of risk modification. This requires specific structural and procedural changes to be implemented, with an educational process for all involved.
- *Integration and support.* Once changes and interventions are decided upon, a system for monitoring their integration into the maternity services is needed to determine if the change has actually reduced or modified the identified risk. The data collection, analysis, measurement, monitoring and re-evaluation constitute the third part of risk modification.

Clinical risk modification is the changing of circumstances, environment and behaviour in order to lower the potential for risk. The result should be improved clinical outcomes and patient satisfaction; the documentation of care should also improve. A proactive risk modification process enables managers and the multidisciplinary team to control effectively the safety, activity, cost and quality of health care.

Picking up the pieces

It is hoped that the tone of this chapter will give the reader cause to be optimistic. There is much that practitioners can do, on an individual basis and as members of an organization, to improve standards. It is, however, only right to acknowledge that perfection cannot be guaranteed. The contemporary emphasis on pregnancy and labour being normal life events is quite correct, but all practitioners are aware that outcomes are sometimes poor, and that very often this is not because anyone has done anything wrong. Paradoxically, the belief in pregnancy's essential normality may have contributed to the expectation that every labour will result in a healthy smiling baby and a happy mother. However, no matter how well planned a clinical risk management strategy is, it will not be able to prevent every poor outcome. Practitioners, then, must be able to deal with adverse healthcare events.

This chapter's earlier section on communication stressed its importance in building up a trusting relationship between a woman and the midwife or doctor. The most severe test of this relationship is likely to come if there is a poor outcome. The feeling of loss, disenchantment or pain may make the woman and her family distrustful. The feeling of a lack of control may make communication especially difficult.

The sensitivity of practitioners at this time is crucial. A midwife's demeanour, and the way in which he or she approaches the woman and her family, may be critical in determining how they respond. In Chapter 10, Thomas and Tansley claim that the failure to acknowledge mistakes, or the perception that staff are dismissive or are withholding information, may even drive people towards litigation. Consumer programmes have alerted people to their rights to complain, and have reinforced the compensation message. Adequate care may count for little if the explanation of a poor outcome is handled without tact and sensitivity. The key to this aspect of risk management, as in so many other areas, is effective communication.

Conclusion

This book has detailed areas in which clinical risk management is important for midwives. While certain areas may already have been familiar to some, the range covered here will have provided new insights for most, if not all, readers.

It will have become obvious that there is no right to a perfect baby. Rights that are not enforceable are worth little; there is so much in pregnancy (as in life) that cannot be predicted or controlled, and little will be gained from demanding perfection. What people have rightly come to expect is that healthcare practitioners will be competent, polite and caring. Clinical risk management can help to promote competence in clinical matters; it can encourage practitioners to respect the autonomy and dignity of those who use the health service; and it can educate clinicians to deal with poor outcomes with prudence and tact. This much is achievable, and is the right of every pregnant woman.

References

Acheson, D. (1991). Are obstetrics and midwifery doomed? *Midwives' Chronicle*, **104**, 158–66.

Anon (2000). Midwife struck off. *Practising Midwife*, **3(5)**, 7.

Bogle, I. (2000). Wanted – examples of good practice. *Br. Med. Assoc. News Rev.*, **Oct**, 33.

Bridges, G. (1999). The public seem to expect their politicians to disinfect the nation's kitchen surfaces. *The Times*, 28 January, p. 22.

Chaston, I. (1994). A comparative study of internal customer management practices within service sector firms and the National Health Service. *J. Adv. Nursing*, **19**, 299–305.

Clyne, M. E. and Forlenza, M. (1997). Consumer-focused preadmission testing: a paradigm shift. *J. Nursing Care Quality*, **11(3)**, 9–15.

Department of Health (1997). *A First Class Service: Quality in the New NHS*. HMSO.

Ellis, J. (1988). Doctors in training: who bears the cost? In: *Medical Negligence: Addressing the Issues*, pp. 8–14. Medical Protection Society.

Henderson, L., Kitzinger, J. and Green, J. (2000). Representing infant feeding: content analysis of British media portrayals of bottle feeding and breast feeding. *Br. Med. J.*, **321**, 1196–8.

Huntingford, P. (1990). Obstetrics and gynaecology. In: *Medical Negligence* (J. Powers and N. Harris, eds). Butterworths.

MMI Companies Inc. (1998). *Transforming Insights into Clinical Practice Improvements: A 12-Year Data Summary Resource*. MMI Companies Inc.

Moore, W. (2000). *Why Doctors Make Mistakes*. Channel 4 Books.

National Audit Office (2001). *Handling Clinical Negligence Claims in England*. HC 403. HMSO.

Rogers, L. (1999). Blunders by doctors kill 40 000 a year. *Sunday Times*, 19 December.

Royal College of Obstetricians and Gynaecologists (2000). *Clinical Risk Management for Obstetricians and Gynaecologists* (Clinical Governance Advice No.2). RCOG Press.

Symon, A. (2001). *Obstetric Litigation from A–Z*. Quay Books.

Taylor-Adams, S. and Lyons, D. (1998). Do obstetric staff know when to call for assistance. *Healthcare Risk Resource*, **1(4)**, 2–3.

United Kingdom Central Council for Nursing, Midwifery and Health Visiting (1996). *Guidelines for Professional Practice*. UKCC.

Walters, D. (2000). *How to Reflect on your Practice. MIDIRS Midwifery Digest*, **10,** 136.

Wilson, J. (1996). *Integrated Care Management: The Path to Success*. Butterworth-Heinemann.

Wilson, J. H. (1997). The Clinical Negligence Scheme for Trusts. *Br. J. Nursing*, **6(20)**, 1166–7.

Index